AF380500

# Practical Controversies in Medical Management of Stone Disease

*Editors*
Margaret S. Pearle
Department of Urology
University of Texas Southwestern
Medical Center
Dallas
Texas, USA

Stephen Y. Nakada
Department of Urology
University of Wisconsin School
of Medicine and Public Health
Madison
Wisconsin, USA

ISBN 978-1-4614-9574-1          ISBN 978-1-4614-9575-8 (eBook)
DOI 10.1007/978-1-4614-9575-8
Springer New York Heidelberg Dordrecht London

Library of Congress Control Number: 2014930307

© Springer Science+Business Media New York 2014
This work is subject to copyright. All rights are reserved by the Publisher, whether the whole or part of the material is concerned, specifically the rights of translation, reprinting, reuse of illustrations, recitation, broadcasting, reproduction on microfilms or in any other physical way, and transmission or information storage and retrieval, electronic adaptation, computer software, or by similar or dissimilar methodology now known or hereafter developed. Exempted from this legal reservation are brief excerpts in connection with reviews or scholarly analysis or material supplied specifically for the purpose of being entered and executed on a computer system, for exclusive use by the purchaser of the work. Duplication of this publication or parts thereof is permitted only under the provisions of the Copyright Law of the Publisher's location, in its current version, and permission for use must always be obtained from Springer. Permissions for use may be obtained through RightsLink at the Copyright Clearance Center. Violations are liable to prosecution under the respective Copyright Law.
The use of general descriptive names, registered names, trademarks, service marks, etc. in this publication does not imply, even in the absence of a specific statement, that such names are exempt from the relevant protective laws and regulations and therefore free for general use.
While the advice and information in this book are believed to be true and accurate at the date of publication, neither the authors nor the editors nor the publisher can accept any legal responsibility for any errors or omissions that may be made. The publisher makes no warranty, express or implied, with respect to the material contained herein.

Printed on acid-free paper

Springer is part of Springer Science+Business Media (www.springer.com)

Margaret S. Pearle • Stephen Y. Nakada
Editors

# Practical Controversies in Medical Management of Stone Disease

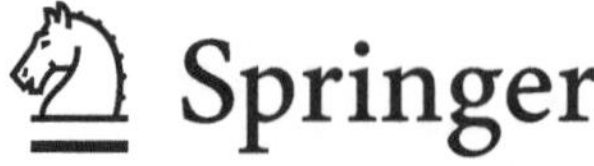 Springer

# Preface

*Practical Controversies in Medical Management of Stone Disease* is targeted at the practitioner interested in caring for patients with kidney stones. Kidney stone disease is a common condition, affecting nearly 1 in 11 individuals in the USA at some time in their lives. Furthermore, the risk of developing a stone does not disappear with passage or treatment of the stone, as recurrence rates for those who have had a stone approach 50 % at 5 years. Consequently, strategies aimed at stone prevention are desirable. Although the literature is replete with books and articles outlining management approaches for stone prevention, there are many areas of disagreement over treatment recommendations, even among stone experts. This book focuses on controversial or misunderstood aspects of evaluation, diet therapy, and medical treatment of stone patients. In each chapter, an expert in the field presents and synthesizes the evidence on a topic from the literature and translates the information into rational treatment recommendations. The aim of this book is to dispel commonly held but incorrect notions about stone disease and to highlight areas ripe for further study. As such, this book will benefit all stakeholders in stones disease, both patients and those caring for them.

Margaret S. Pearle

Stephen Y. Nakada

# Contents

# Contributors

**Jodi Antonelli** Department of Urology, University of Texas Southwestern Medical Center, Dallas, USA

**Sara L. Best** Department of Urology, University of Wisconsin School of Medicine and Public Health, Madison, USA

**Juan C. Calle** Department of Nephrology and Hypertension, Cleveland Clinic, Cleveland, USA

**Brian H. Eisner** Department of Urology, Massachusetts General Hospital, GRB 1102, Boston, USA

**David S. Goldfarb** Nephrology, New York Harbor VA Healthcare System, NYU Langone Medical Center, New York, USA

**Gautam Jayram** The Johns Hopkins Hospital, James Buchanan Brady Urological Institute, Baltimore, USA

**John J. Knoedler** Department of Urology, Mayo Clinic, Rochester, USA

**Amy E. Krambeck** Department of Urology, Mayo Clinic, Rochester, USA

**Michael P. Kurtz** Department of Urology, Massachusetts General Hospital, GRB 1102, Boston, USA

**Michael E. Lipkin** Comprehensive Kidney Stone Center, Urology Division, Surgery Department, Duke University Medical Center, Durham, USA

**Brian R. Matlaga** The Johns Hopkins Hospital, James Buchanan Brady Urological Institute, Baltimore, USA

**Manoj Monga** Stevan Streem Center of Endourology and Stone Disease, Cleveland Clinic, Cleveland, USA

**Margaret S. Pearle** Department of Urology, University of Texas Southwestern Medical Center, Dallas, USA

**Kristina L. Penniston** Department of Urology, University of Wisconsin School of Medicine and Public Health, Madison, USA

**Glenn M. Preminger** Comprehensive Kidney Stone Center, Urology Division, Surgery Department, Duke University Medical Center, Durham, USA

**Khashayar Sakhaee** Charles and Jane Pak Center for Mineral Metabolism and Clinical Research, University of Texas Soutwestern Medical Center, Dallas, USA

**Nicola T. Sumorok** Medical Service, New York Harbor VA Healthcare System, NYU Langone Medical Center, New York, USA

**Ramy F. Youssef** Comprehensive Kidney Stone Center, Urology Division, Surgery Department, Duke University Medical Center, Durham, USA

# Chapter 1
# Metabolic Evaluation: Underused or Overdone?

Juan C. Calle and Manoj Monga

## Introduction

Urolithiasis is a very common clinical problem that places a heavy economic burden on society and has serious effects on the quality of life [1]. It affects both men and women with lifetime prevalence as high as 13 and 7 %, respectively [2]. Over the past few decades, it has been shown that the incidence and prevalence of nephrolithiasis has steadily increased. This is attributed presumably to multiple factors including, but not limited to, changes in diet and lifestyle, increments in the prevalence of obesity and diabetes mellitus, which have also been associated with the formation of kidney stones, migration from rural cooler settings to warmer urban areas, and even possible changes associated to global warming [3, 4]. With this rising prevalence, an increased emphasis has been placed on identifying effective approaches to stone prevention.

The importance of appropriate management of kidney stone disease is underscored by the high incidence of recurrence of the disease after a first episode. Multiple studies have demonstrated that up to 50 % of patients may present with another episode within 5 years of the first kidney stone [5]. When the follow-up period is extended 25 years beyond the incident of stone event, up to 100 % recurrence has been reported [6, 7].

With more than 2 million emergency room visits per year due to renal colic or renal calculus, this ailment represents a massive burden to the health care system and the economy as a whole. The annual direct costs calculated based on data from a private insured, employed population during the year 2000 surpassed US\$ 4.5 billion. After

J. C. Calle (✉)
Department of Nephrology and Hypertension, Cleveland Clinic, 9500 Euclid Avenue, Cleveland, OH 44195, USA
e-mail: callej@ccf.org

M. Monga
Stevan Streem Center of Endourology and Stone Disease, Cleveland Clinic, Q10-1 9500 Euclid Avenue,Cleveland, OH 44195, USA
e-mail: mongam@ccf.org

M. S. Pearle, S. Y. Nakada (eds.), *Practical Controversies in Medical Management of Stone Disease,* DOI 10.1007/978-1-4614-9575-8_1,
© Springer Science+Business Media New York 2014

conservative estimates for indirect costs such as workdays lost due to the disease were calculated, the total projected economic burden increased to more than US$ 5.3 billion [8]. In addition, recent data suggest that kidney stone disease can have significant impact on renal function, cardiovascular risks, psychological distress, and quality of life [9]. In this chapter, we will focus on the role of a metabolic evaluation in the evaluation, management, and follow-up of patients with kidney stone disease.

## General Evaluation

A detailed history from the patient is important to elicit certain medical conditions, dietary habits, medications, past medical history, family history, and social history that may predispose to stone disease.

Common systemic conditions have been associated with stone disease. Hypertension, diabetes, and obesity regarded as part of the metabolic syndrome have been linked to an increased risk of uric acid kidney stones [10, 11]. Gastrointestinal abnormalities such as intestinal resections, bariatric surgery, and chronic diarrhea usually in the setting of inflammatory bowel disease may predispose patients through various pathological mechanisms to certain types of kidney stones, often linked to low urine volume, hypocitraturia, and/or hyperoxaluria [10, 12]. Bone mineral disorders mostly associated with hyperparathyroidism increase the risk of calcium phosphate stones and have also been associated with nephrocalcinosis [13]. Sarcoidosis is associated with stone disease via abnormalities in the calcium-phosphorus-vitamin D axis [14]. Acid-base disorders, more specifically distal renal tubular acidosis alone or as a manifestation of systemic illnesses such as Sjögren syndrome, and other tubulointerstitial nephritis are associated with renal stones [15].

It is also of importance to know the patient's current and past medications, herbal and vitamin supplementations. Agents such as protease inhibitors for the treatment of HIV, topiramate, acetazolamide, triamterene, vitamin C, and calcium supplements in certain conditions may increase the risk of formation and recurrence of kidney stones [16, 17].

## Laboratory Evaluation

There is still much controversy as to whether or not a complete metabolic evaluation should be conducted in all patients who present with a first kidney stone. Regardless of this, and even though the most recent US Preventive Services Task Force concluded that "there is not enough evidence to determine the potential benefits and harms of screening all adults for chronic kidney disease (CKD)" [18], based on our experience and expert opinion, we recommend to obtain serum chemistries including baseline kidney function, serum electrolytes (including calcium and phosphorus), and uric acid for all patients. Urine analysis (UA) should include both dipstick and microscopy. Specific gravity, pH, blood cells, bacteria, and specific crystals may help to clarify the etiology of the stone. Urine culture should be obtained when indicated by findings in the UA, clinical presentation or history of recurrent urinary tract infections (UTI). The presence of urea-splitting bacteria is suggestive of struvite stones [19]. Intact parathyroid hormone (iPTH) should be obtained as part of the screening evaluation if primary hyperparathyroidism is suspected (e.g., symptoms elicited during interrogation consistent with this disease, when serum calcium is high or borderline high and phosphorus is low or borderline low). Also, it should be part of the regular follow-up when the stone is formed predominantly of calcium phosphate, when there is marked hypercalciuria in the absence of elevated urinary sodium levels, or when imaging support findings of nephrocalcinosis [20]. 25-hydroxy-vitamin D should be ordered when calcium abnormalities and iPTH are found [19]. Rare cases of nephrocalcinosis due to vitamin D intoxication have also been described in the literature [21].

## 24-h Urine Collections

This is perhaps the most controversial topic in the testing of patients with kidney stone disease due to conflicting results available in the literature and the dearth of well-designed randomized controlled trials. Based on earlier literature and reports showing a high recurrence of stone formation after a first-time event, and the high morbidity and costs associated with it, some authorities recommend a full metabolic workup including a 24-h urine collection in all stone formers [22]. On the other hand, there are data to support the recommendation not to obtain 24-h urine collections on all first-time stone formers and reserve this evaluation only for recurrent stone formers [23] or those with other known risk factors such as recommended by the European Association of Urology [24]. Various studies have also shown evidence that comprehensive medical evaluation and treatment associated with the results of these thorough investigations offered no advantage in cost or efficacy over empiric treatment [25, 26]. However, these results may be dependent on international variations in medical practice and medical cost and insurance coverage differences [27].

In general, patients who are highly motivated to change dietary and health habits, those with single kidneys, those with multiple stones or stone episodes, and subjects with multiple and severe comorbidities should be offered a full metabolic evaluation. A small retrospective study by Krambeck et al. demonstrated at least one abnormal metabolic finding in all of the patients with known calcium phosphate (brushite) stones ($n=45$) in whom 24-h metabolic urine collections were available [28]. Hence, we recommend that these individuals should also have a more extensive and complete evaluation. By the same principle and as mentioned above, those patients with other known high risks for recurrence of stone formation such as gastrointestinal diseases with chronic diarrhea and malabsorption, bariatric surgery, genetically associated stone formation, drugs linked to stone formation, and anatomical conditions that make patients prone to stone recurrence should also undergo a complete metabolic evaluation.

Once the controversy of whether to obtain a 24-h urine collection is addressed, it is followed closely by the controversy of obtaining only one collection versus more than one collection. Previous studies by Pak et al. have demonstrated that only one 24-h collection provides reliable information for the management of patients with kidney stone disease [29], and most studies have corroborated these findings [30]. Other investigators have reported significant variation in results that can impact management plans, suggesting that two 24-h urine collections are needed to appropriately and accurately guide the therapy [31–33]. However, the costs and burden on the patients for the collection should be taken in consideration and have been mentioned as limiting factors by these investigators. It is interesting to note that all of these are retrospective studies. One may speculate that differences in geographical and seasonal changes that have not been analyzed in these studies may have played a role in the opposing results as evidenced by the concordant findings in the studies from southern geographical locations [29, 30] compared to the northern geographical locations [31–33].

The analysis of the 24-h urine collections should include urine volume, calcium, oxalate, phosphate, urate, sodium, potassium, and pH. In specific cases when cystine stones or cystinuria is suspected or known to be the etiology of the disease, measurement of 24-h urine cystine should be completed. For patients found to have hypercalciuria, there is no evidence to support additional historical testing (fasting, calcium load) to differentiate the type of hypercalciuria (absorptive type 1 or 2, renal), as these distinctions have not been shown to afford any clinical advantage [34, 35]. Supersaturation studies can also be performed when available as these have been found to be predictive of recurrence of the disease, and stone composition correlates fairly well with urinary supersaturation [36]. We do not recommend spot urine collections given the high variability of results dependent on dietary and fluid intake at any given time [37].

In the most recent comparative effectiveness review by the Agency for Health Care Research and Quality in the USA, it was confirmed that no high-quality randomized control trials were identified to assess outcomes between treatments for subgroups stratified by baseline biochemistry levels or 24-h urine collections. Also, there was little evidence that baseline urine calcium and oxalate levels (together the most common type of kidney stones) predicted response to different therapeutic approaches including fluid intake, diet, thiazides, or citrate versus control on recurrent stone outcomes. It is also worth mentioning that in the same report there was no good evidence from randomized control trials to support whether follow-up blood and urine biochemistry measurements predict final health outcomes and intermediate stone outcomes [38].

## Stone Composition Analysis

Stone composition should be determined when available, as this may help to uncover metabolic disorders and pathophysiology of stone formers, especially in unusual diseases such as cystinuria, adenine phosphoribosyltransferase deficiency, xanthine stones, and crystallization of drugs. Stone composition may direct future medical management, specifically for uric acid, struvite, and cystine stone formers. Furthermore, it may provide urologists with information necessary to choose between different endourological treatment options [39]. The analysis is usually performed by X-ray crystallography or infrared spectroscopy, but other techniques such as direct chemical analysis, polarization microscopy, thermogravimetry, and scanning electron microscopy can also be used. However, each of them may have different limitations in terms of cost, the need for relatively large amounts of sample and even the differentiation of some components [40].

## Conclusion

In this review, we outline the importance of a detailed and thorough history for patients with kidney stones. Whether a full metabolic workup is needed for all first-time patients with a kidney stone is still controversial, and there are no conclusive available data from randomized controlled trials. Nonetheless, all patients should have basic serum chemistries and urine analysis. Twenty-four-hour metabolic urine collections seem to be appropriate for patients with recurrent stone disease or those with complicated medical histories, although once more, more data from well-designed studies are needed. Stone composition should always be performed when available.

## References


1. Lotan Y. Economics and cost of care of stone disease. Adv Chronic Kidney Dis. 2009;16(1):5–10
2. Stamatelou KK, Francis ME, Jones CA, Nyberg LM, Curhan GC, et al. Time trends in reported prevalence of kidney stones in the United States: 1976–1994. Kidney Int. 2003;63(5):1817–23.
3. Lieske JC, Peña de la Vega LS, Slezak JM, Bergstralh EJ, Leibson CL, Ho KL, et al. Renal stone epidemiology in Rochester, Minnesota: an update. Kidney Int. 2006;69(4):760–4.
4. Taylor EN, Stampfer MJ, Curhan GC. Obesity, weight gain, and the risk of kidney stones. J Am Med Assoc. 2005;293:455–62.
5. Hall PM. Nephrolithiasis: treatment, causes, and prevention. Cleve Clin J Med. 2009;76(10):583–91.
6. Coe FL, Keck J, Norton ER. The natural history of calcium urolithiasis. J Am Med Assoc. 1977;238(14):1519–23.
7. Williams RE. Long-term survey of 538 patients with upper urinary tract stone. Br J Urol. 1963;35:416–37.
8. Saigal CS, Joyce G, Timilsina AR. Direct and indirect costs of nephrolithiasis in an employed population: opportunity for disease management? Kidney Int. 2005 Oct;68(4):1808–14
9. Kartha G, Calle JC, Marchini GS, Monga M. Impact of stone disease: chronic kidney disease and quality of life. Urol Clin North Am. 2013 Feb;40(1):135–47.
10. Sakhaee K, Maalouf NM, Sinnott B. Kidney stones 2012: pathogenesis, diagnosis, and management. J Clin Endocrinol Metab. 2012;97:1847–60.
11. Maalouf NM. Metabolic syndrome and the genesis of uric acid stones. J Ren Nutr. 2011;21:128–31.
12. Lieske JC, Kumar R, Collazo-Clavell ML. Nephrolithiasis after bariatric surgery for obesity. Semin Nephrol. 2008 Mar;28(2):163–73.
13. Suh JM, Cronan JJ, Monchik JM. Primary hyperparathyroidism: is there an increased prevalence of renal stone disease? Am J Roentgenol. 2008 Sep;191(3):908–11.
14. Casella FJ, Allon M. The kidney in sarcoidosis. J Am Soc Nephrol. 1993 Mar;3(9):1555–62.

15. Buckalew VM Jr. Nephrolithiasis in renal tubular acidosis. J Urol.1989 Mar; 141(3 Pt 2):731–7.
16. Daudon M, Jungers P. Drug-induced renal calculi: epidemiology, prevention and management. Drugs 2004;64:245–75.
17. Curhan GC, Willett WC, Rimm EB, Stampfer MJ. A prospective study of the intake of vitamins C and B6, and the risk of kidney stones in men. J Urol 1996;155:1847–51.
18. U.S. Preventive Services Task Force. 2013. http://www.uspreventiveservicestaskforce.org. Accessed May 2013.
19. Goldfarb DS, Arowojolu O. Metabolic evaluation of first-time and recurrent stone formers. Urol Clin North Am. 2013 Feb;40(1):13–20.
20. Peacock M. Primary hyperparathyroidism and the kidney: biochemical and clinical spectrum. J Bone Miner Res. 2002 Nov;17(Suppl 2):N87–94.
21. Beşbaş N, Oner A, Akhan O, Saatçi U, Bakkaloğlu A, Topaloğlu R. Nephrocalcinosis due to vitamin D intoxication. Turk J Pediatr. 1989 Jul-Sep;31(3):239–44.
22. Parmar MS. Kidney stones. BMJ. 2004 Jun 12;328(7453):1420–4.
23. Goldfarb DS. Reconsideration of the 1988 NIH Consensus Statement on Prevention and Treatment of Kidney Stones: are the recommendations out of date? Rev Urol. 2002 Spring;4(2):53–60.
24. Turk C, Knoll T, Petrik A, Sarica K, Skolarikos A, Straub M, Seitz C. Guidelines on Urolithiasis. 2013. http://www.uroweb.org/gls/pdf/21_Urolithiasis_LR.pdf. Accessed May 2013.
25. Chandhoke PS. When is medical prophylaxis cost-effective for recurrent calcium stones? J Urol. 2002 Sep;168(3):937–40.
26. Lotan Y, Cadeddu JA, Roerhborn CG, Pak CY, Pearle MS. Cost-effectiveness of medical management strategies for nephrolithiasis. J Urol. 2004 Dec; 172(6 Pt 1):2275–81.
27. Lotan Y, Cadeddu JA, Pearle MS. International comparison of cost effectiveness of medical management strategies for nephrolithiasis. Urol Res. 2005 Jun;33(3):223–30.
28. Krambeck AE, Handa SE, Evan AP, Lingeman JE. Profile of the brushite stone former. J Urol. 2010 Oct;184(4):1367–71.
29. Pak CY, Peterson R, Poindexter JR. Adequacy of a single stone risk analysis in the medical evaluation of urolithiasis. J Urol. 2001 Feb;165(2):378–81.
30. Castle SM, Cooperberg MR, Sadetsky N, Eisner BH, Stoller ML. Adequacy of a single 24-hour urine collection for metabolic evaluation of recurrent nephrolithiasis. J Urol. 2010 Aug;184(2):579–83.
31. Parks JH, Goldfisher E, Asplin JR, Coe FL. A single 24-hour urine collection is inadequate for the medical evaluation of nephrolithiasis. J Urol. 2002 Apr;167(4):1607–12.
32. Healy KA, Hubosky SG, Bagley D. 24-Hour urine collection in the metabolic evaluation of stone formers: Is one study adequate? J Endourol. 2013 Mar;27(3):374–8.
33. Nayan M, Elkoushy MA, Andonian S. Variations between two 24-hour urine collections in patients presenting to a tertiary stone clinic. Can Urol Assoc J. 2012 Feb;6(1):30–3.
34. Lein JW, Keane PM. Limitations of the oral calcium loading test in the management of the recurrent calcareous renal stone former. Am J Kidney Dis. 1983;3(1):76–9.
35. Pak CY, Sakhaee K, Pearle MS. Detection of absorptive hypercalciuria type I without the oral calcium load test. J Urol. 2011;185(3):915–9.
36. Coe FL, Wise H, Parks JH, Asplin JR: Proportional reduction of urine supersaturation during nephrolithiasis treatment. J Urol. 2001;166(4):1247–51.
37. Hong YH, Dublin N, Razack AH, Mohd MA, Husain R. Twenty-four hour and spot urine metabolic evaluations: correlations versus agreements. Urology. 2010 Jun;75(6):1294–8.
38. Fink HA, Wilt TJ, Eidman KE, Garimella PS, MacDonald R, Rutks IR, et al. Recurrent nephrolithiasis in adults: comparative effectiveness of preventive medical strategies [Internet]. Comparative Effectiveness Review No. 61. Report No.: 12-EHC049–EF. Rockville: Agency for Healthcare Research and Quality (US); 2012.
39. Kijvikai K, de la Rosette JJ. Assessment of stone composition in the management of urinary stones. Nat Rev Urol. 2011 Feb;8(2):81–5.
40. Basiri A, Taheri M, Taheri F. What is the state of the stone analysis techniques in urolithiasis? Urol J. 2012 Spring;9(2):445–54.

# Chapter 2
# Dietary oxalate and calcium oxalate stones: a theoretical or real concern?

Kristina L. Penniston

## Introduction

Oxalic acid is the simplest and most acidic of the dicarboxylic organic acids (Fig. 2.1). It is used commercially in rust removal, cleaning, and bleaching formulations. The beekeeping industry in Europe and Canada utilizes oxalic acid dihydrate against varroa, parasitic mites that prey on honey bees [1]. Additionally, oxalate-containing products are currently being investigated for therapeutic potential as dental desensitizing agents [2]. Oxalate (IUPAC name, ethanedioate), the conjugated anion of the acid, forms salts with cations such as calcium, magnesium, iron, zinc, sodium, and potassium. These salts vary greatly with respect to solubility, with sodium and potassium oxalates being soluble, and magnesium, calcium, zinc, iron, and other cations forming less soluble to virtually insoluble oxalate compounds.

## *Oxalate in the Environment*

Oxalate in many forms is widely distributed in nature. Calcium oxalates (whewellite and weddellite) form the scialbatura or "crust" on weathered buildings and monuments [3]. Calcium oxalate residues on rock surfaces, produced and deposited by epithelial lichen, are used in radiocarbon dating and in paleoclimate reconstruction [4]. Oxalic acid is produced by certain fungi and algae. Oxalic acid production by pathogenic fungal strains, such as *Aspergillus* and *Penicillium*, apparently plays a role in their pathogenic capabilities [5]. In algae, which typically subsist in mineral-rich oceanic environments, oxalic acid production is thought to serve as a mineral detoxification mechanism as well as protection against herbivory [6]. The potential

K. L. Penniston (✉)
Department of Urology, University of Wisconsin School of Medicine and Public Health,
1685 Highland Avenue, 3258 MFCB,
Madison, WI 53705-2281, USA
e-mail: penn@urology.wisc.edu

M. S. Pearle, S. Y. Nakada (eds.), *Practical Controversies in Medical Management of Stone Disease,* DOI 10.1007/978-1-4614-9575-8_2,
© Springer Science+Business Media New York 2014

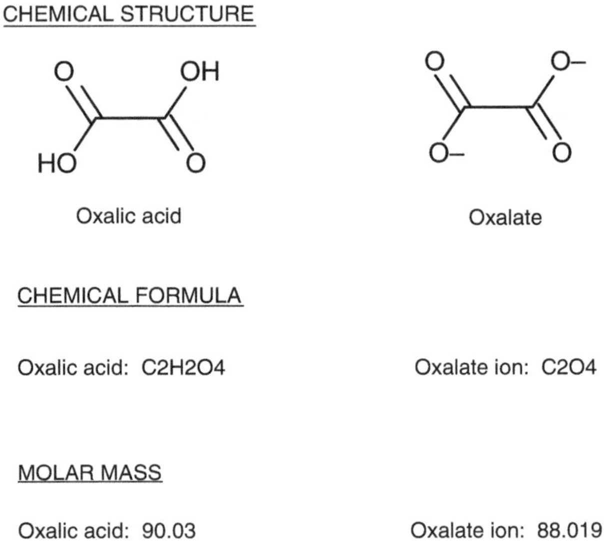

**Fig. 2.1** Chemical structure, formula, and molar mass of oxalic acid and oxalate, its conjugated anion

CHEMICAL STRUCTURE

Oxalic acid

Oxalate

CHEMICAL FORMULA

Oxalic acid: $C_2H_2O_4$

Oxalate ion: $C_2O_4$

MOLAR MASS

Oxalic acid: 90.03

Oxalate ion: 88.019

of soil as a long-term sink of atmospheric carbon dioxide is currently being studied and would potentially include the use and management of oxalogenic plants and oxalotrophic bacteria in a process known as the oxalate-carbonate pathway [7].

## Oxalate in Plants

Calcium oxalate is also found in rocks and calcareous sediments [8]. Oxalate in various forms is taken up ubiquitously by most vascular plants, which exploit the calcium-binding potential of oxalate primarily to regulate intracellular pH and calcium concentrations but also, as in the case of plants with crystalliferous cells, as a feeding deterrent against certain insects [9]. Gravity perception and mechanical support are also theorized functions for calcium oxalate complexation [10], as is the mineral-chelating property of oxalate to protect against toxicity [5, 11].

Plants also synthesize oxalate via oxidation of glycolate and glyoxylate and, in some cases, ascorbic acid. Certain plants have extremely high amounts of oxalate; these include those in the *Oxalis* genus of the Oxalidaceae family (e.g., various wood sorrels, oca tubers), members of the Cactaceae family, and more commonly consumed plants such as fat hen or "lamb's quarters," rhubarb leaves (the oxalate content of the stalk comprises only about 2 % of the total acidity), buckwheat grain, star fruit, spinach, beet greens (beet roots have less oxalate), and some nuts, (e.g., almonds, cashews) [12]. A comprehensive list of the oxalate content of commonly consumed foods, analyzed with modern instrumentation, is available online [13]. A table of some commonly consumed foods is provided (Table 2.1). The bioavailability in humans of the oxalate in these and other foods is highly dependent on the predominant salt forms of oxalate and on other constituents of the meal in which the

**Table 2.1** Commonly consumed foods that are reportedly high in oxalate[a]

| Food | Serving size | Oxalate/serving (mg) |
| --- | --- | --- |
| Spinach, cooked | 1/2 cup | 755 |
| Spinach, raw | 1 cup | 656 |
| Rhubarb | 1/2 cup | 541 |
| Almonds | 1 ounce (about 22 nuts) | 122 |
| Wheat berries, cooked | 1 cup | 98 |
| Baked potato, with skin | 1 medium | 97 |
| Corn grits | 1 cup | 97 |
| Bulgur, cooked | 1 cup | 86 |
| Beets | 1/2 cup | 76 |
| Navy beans | 1/2 cup | 76 |
| Hot chocolate (homemade) | 1 cup | 65 |
| Okra | 1/2 cup | 57 |
| Shredded wheat and bran cereal | 1–1/4 cup | 53 |
| French fries | 4 ounces (about 1/2 cup) | 51 |
| Cashews | 1 ounce (about 18 nuts) | 49 |
| Raspberries | 1 cup | 48 |
| Raisin bran cereal | 1 cup | 46 |
| Lentil soup | 1 cup | 39 |
| Chocolate syrup | 2 tablespoons | 38 |
| Multi-bran chex cereal | 1 cup | 36 |

[a] Cooking and/or preparation method is listed if provided; see [13]

food is consumed. Thus, the oxalate content of a food or meal may have less clinical relevance than oxalate bioavailability.

## *Oxalate in Humans*

While oxalate has long been associated with urolithiasis and oxalosis in humans and animals, it is increasingly gaining attention in other medical conditions in which it is theorized to play a role, in some scenarios, independent of its renal handling. These include pancreatitis/exocrine pancreatic insufficiency [14], autism, vulvar pain, and in cases of coronary atherosclerosis [15].

## **Background**

In the USA and in other modern nations, calcium oxalate is the predominant complex of most urinary tract stones. Calcium and oxalate both appear normally in urine. Calcium is normally excreted over a 24-h period in the range of 50–250 mg, depending on gender, body size, diet, and other factors [16]. Calcium is tightly regulated in the body with only 1 % of the total body store in circulation under normal physiologic conditions. Approximately 15–25 % of the calcium ingested on a balanced diet is excreted in urine, but many factors affect it [17]. Urine oxalate, on the other hand, is derived from the ingestion of foods that contain it and its precursors (e.g., ascorbic acid, hydroxyproline) and also from hepatic biosynthesis, as oxalate is an end product of several metabolic pathways involving amino acids, carbohydrates, and ascorbic acid [18]. Early research presumed that urinary oxalate excretion was primarily from exogenous sources [19]. But the intake of oxalate or its precursors is now known to account for 10–50 % of 24-h urinary oxalate excretion, depending on other dietary factors and gut physiology and transport [20, 21]. Endogenous production is the remaining source of urinary oxalate.

## Intake and Metabolism of Oxalate

Oxalate is a phytochemical obtained nearly exclusively from plant foods. Phytochemicals are nonnutritive plant compounds and include carotenoids, polyphenols, flavonoids, and other antioxidants, many of which confer health benefits [22]. Oxalate, while a phytochemical, is not known for any health benefit to humans. In fact, it is commonly referred to as an "anti-nutrient" for its ability to bind with calcium, magnesium, zinc, iron, and other cations in the gastrointestinal tract and reduce their absorption [23], potentially leading to mineral deficiency. It has been known since the turn of the twentieth century that oxalate absorption is reduced when complexed with calcium [24]. Long before understanding a mechanism, practitioners in ancient Mesopotamia (between 3200 and 1200 BC) advised ostrich egg shells, rich in calcium, as treatment for urinary tract stones [25], presumably as a binder of lithogenic promoters in urine.

Because humans and most animals lack the enzymatic capacity to metabolize oxalate, excretion is necessary to avoid pathological consequences from high circulating oxalate. Depending on overall plant intake, and more directly on the intake of certain plants, human intake ranges from negligible amounts to as much or more than 1,000 mg per day [18, 26]. In the USA, oxalate intake is estimated to average 150–200 mg per day [27, 28].

## Urine Supersaturation of Calcium Oxalate

Many individuals, including non-stone formers, have a relative supersaturation of calcium oxalate in their urine [29]. Calcium oxalate crystals are thus thought to form frequently but then to pass in urine without symptoms or pathological consequences. Individuals whose urinary calcium and oxalate concentrations are within the normal ranges can form calcium oxalate stones if urine volume is low enough and/or if there are perturbations in other urinary parameters. Renal calcium oxalate crystal formation and growth is inhibited by various indigenous urinary factors, and the relative presence or lack of these is thought to account for the fact that calcium oxalate kidney stone prevalence is only about 13–15 % in the USA [30], when, in fact, most individuals form calcium oxalate crystals.

## *Prevalence of High Urine Oxalate*

High urinary oxalate excretion is a major risk factor for calcium oxalate stones. Urine oxalate is generally considered within a normal range if it is less than 40 mg in a 24-h period, though, with respect to calcium oxalate stone risk, less urinary oxalate excretion is desirable; an upper limit of 30 mg per day has been suggested [31, 32]. The reported range of 24-h urinary oxalate in non-stone forming humans is 10–40 mg. The prevalence of high urinary oxalate excretion among idiopathic calcium oxalate stone formers ranges widely between 15 and 50 % [31], suggesting that other mechanisms of stone formation are responsible in the majority of calcium oxalate stone formers (excluding those with one of the primary hyperoxalurias). Its incidence is higher among individuals with gastrointestinal malabsorption and enteric hyperoxaluria [33]. It is also high in individuals whose calcium intake is lower than recommended, typically about 1,000 mg/day for most adults [31]. There are reports of seasonal variability of oxalate excretion [34, 35], and the intake of oxalate may not be consistent throughout the week on a day-to-day basis. Thus, the true estimation of hyperoxaluria prevalence in idiopathic stone formers is complicated as over- or underestimation of an individual's relative risk within a given time period may occur depending on the season or day of urine collection.

## *Importance of High Urine Oxalate*

Urinary oxalate excretion is normally between five- and tenfold less than calcium (mg/mg). It is widely held that a minor increase in urinary oxalate can have a substantial lithogenic effect. Calculations of the ratio of gradients for oxalate and calcium, using data for typical urine, have revealed that the rate of change in relative supersaturation is 10–23 times greater for oxalate than calcium [36–39]. For this reason, some argue that urinary oxalate excretion should be considered a continuous, not a dichotomous, variable.

While a small increase in urinary oxalate excretion can significantly increase calcium oxalate stone risk, the presence of high urine oxalate does not account for the majority of calcium oxalate cases (excluding patients with one of the primary hyperoxalurias). Other urinary factors that are therefore important for calcium oxalate stone risk, especially in patients whose 24-h urinary oxalate excretions appear well controlled, include urine volume, as even those with no known risk factors can form oxalate-containing calculi if urine is highly concentrated. Other factors include citrate, which forms a soluble complex with calcium in urine, rendering less calcium available to bind with oxalate. Phytate, though not typically measured by laboratories providing 24-h urine analyses for stone risk, also forms a soluble complex with calcium in urine. Magnesium forms a complex with oxalate, preventing calcium oxalate complexation; the magnesium oxalate complex is about 600 times more soluble in urine than calcium oxalate.

## *Medical and Nutritional Management of High Urine Oxalate*

Currently, there is no pharmacologic agent designed specifically to reduce urinary oxalate concentration, although cholestyramine has been prescribed with reported effect in some cases [40, 41] but not others [42]. Conjugated bile acid replacement is potentially useful in the subset of patients with bile acid malabsorption [43, 44], and pancreatic enzyme therapy may be useful in patients with pancreatic insufficiency associated with fat malabsorption [45]. Herbal and nontraditional remedies have been reviewed [46], but none appear to have the evidence required for widespread adoption in medical management. Some over-the-counter supplements may help reduce urinary oxalate excretion, specifically fish oil containing docosahexanoic acid (DHA) and eicosapentanoic acid (EPA) [47, 48] and pyridoxine (vitamin $B_6$) in supraphysiologic dosages [49, 50].

The mechanisms of action for these agents are not known, but candidate theories involve both oxalate biosynthesis and effects on renal calcium oxalate deposition and retention. Oxalate-degrading plant enzymes, extracted and concentrated from some fruits and vegetables, as well as plant stem extracts, have been proposed to reduce oxalate biosynthesis [51]. But data are limited, especially with respect to dosages and the generalizability of results to idiopathic calcium oxalate stone formers. As many strains of bacteria are known to degrade oxalate [52], probiotic supplements have been promoted as a way to reduce oxalate absorption and thus its urinary excretion. But this, too, has limited supportive data [53, 54], and some data actually show no effect at all [55].

Clinically, oxalate intake from foods and beverages is manipulated with variable reported efficacy on calcium oxalate stone prevention. Medications to control certain urinary risk factors are also employed. All medical strategies to reduce high urine oxalate appear most useful when directed by the patient's specific etiology. Determining the cause of a patient's hyperoxaluria is imperative. Because there is currently variable clinical evidence, controversy surrounds efficacy of the two major approaches: (1) controlling the absorption of exogenous oxalate, and (2) controlling the endogenous production of oxalate. The rationales for currently used strategies within these approaches are reviewed.

## Control the Gastrointestinal Absorption of Oxalate

### *Enhance the Binding of Cations with Oxalate in the Gastrointestinal Tract*

#### Rationale

Oxalate absorption in the gastrointestinal tract can be reduced by dietary means. Strategies are:

1. Increase or optimize intake of cations (there is most support for calcium and magnesium) with high binding affinity for oxalate.
2. Decrease or limit the presence of digestive contents (e.g., fat) that interfere with the availability of cations to bind oxalate.

### *Enhance Gastrointestinal Degradation of Oxalate by Bacteria*

#### Rationale

The lack of oxalate-degrading gut bacteria in stone formers is reported. There are many common gastrointestinal bacteria that consume oxalate to one degree or another. The bacterial profile of the human gut can be manipulated with diet. Strategies are:

1. Increase or optimize intake of bacteria known to degrade oxalate.
2. Increase or optimize colonization and proliferation of oxalate-degrading bacteria by manipulating the intake of prebiotic material.

### *Control Gastrointestinal Concentration of Soluble Oxalate*

#### Rationale

Certain individuals are thought to be "hyperabsorbers" of oxalate, primarily including those with short bowel malabsorption or with underlying malabsorptive conditions (e.g., cystic fibrosis, celiac disease). Strategies for these individuals include:

1. Reduce or otherwise control the intake of soluble oxalate.
2. Reduce or otherwise control bile acid-mediated oxalate absorption in the gastrointestinal tract (low-fat diet, conjugated bile acid therapy).

## Control the Biosynthesis of Oxalate

### *Increase or Optimize Enzymatic Capacity to Reduce Oxalate Biosynthesis*

**Rationale**

The hepatic enzyme L-alanine glyoxylate aminotransferase (AGT) prevents oxalate formation. This enzyme is deficient in patients with primary hyperoxaluria type 1 (PH1). Moreover, individuals with vitamin $B_6$ deficiency may have suboptimal enzyme activity, as vitamin $B_6$ is a cofactor for the enzyme. Strategies are:

1. Combined liver/kidney transplantation (in the case of the primary hyperoxalurias).
2. Supplemental vitamin $B_6$ (pyridoxine), which works for approximately one-third of PH1 patients who are responsive to therapy and for idiopathic calcium oxalate stone formers whose vitamin $B_6$ deficiency is corrected, thereby restoring normal enzyme activity. A role for pyridoxine therapy in the vitamin $B_6$-sufficient idiopathic calcium oxalate stone former is also reported but remains questionable.

### *Reduce or Control Oxalate Substrate Concentration*

**Rationale**

Dietary sources of oxalate substrates have been shown to increase oxalate biosynthesis. Strategies are:

1. Control or limit supplements containing high doses of ascorbic acid.
2. Control or limit intake of foods and supplements providing fructose, hydroxyproline, glycolate, and glycine.

Although the above approaches are commonly incorporated in medical management, there is a lack of consensus about the value and effectiveness of some. Some of the major questions and controversies surrounding the control of high urine oxalate as a risk factor for the idiopathic calcium oxalate stone former are reviewed.

## Controversies and Unanswered Questions Surrounding the Clinical Control of High Urinary Oxalate Excretion

### *Should a Low Oxalate Diet Be Recommended for All Calcium Oxalate Stone Formers?*

- ***Data for broad-sweeping dietary oxalate restriction are lacking.*** There are no controlled studies proving reduced calcium oxalate stone recurrence with a dietary oxalate restriction. The comparative effectiveness of medical management strategies has been reviewed [56] and a low oxalate diet was not shown to be effective. Some studies show reduced urine oxalate with low oxalate diets [57], but others do not, including among patients after Roux-en-Y surgery, whose hyperoxaluria is thought to be especially receptive to oxalate restriction [58]. Epidemiologic work has revealed an unclear relation between oxalate intake and stones [59], and no impact of diet on 24-h urinary oxalate excretion was found [28]. It may be that studies to date have not selected patient subjects appropriately to test the theory that a low oxalate diet can reduce urinary oxalate excretion. Selection of patients for future studies should be aimed at identifying those most likely to benefit from dietary oxalate restriction as it appears not all patients do. Results may then be more conclusive.

- ***Oxalate restriction does not always address the problem.*** A dietary oxalate restriction is clearly not indicated if a patient does not have high urine oxalate (as in ~80% of calcium oxalate stone formers). Restriction in these cases will have no clinical efficacy, and lack of "success" could reduce the patient's enthusiasm for medical management. Moreover, diet restrictions in general are known for their potential to restrict nutrient intake and, in the case of stone formers, may even compromise the expression of urinary stone inhibitors, as the foods they are advised to avoid are often those with the highest concentration of urinary stone inhibitors (e.g., phytate, magnesium, citric acid, antioxidants).

- ***High urine oxalate is infrequently caused by a high oxalate intake.*** One of the largest dietary sources of oxalate in the USA is spinach [59], but its intake may not be widespread. Only 12% of patients in a study that evaluated 4-day diet records from stone patients consumed any spinach at all [60]. Moreover, some of the other notoriously high-oxalate foods are only eaten occasionally by most people, and these include rhubarb and beets. If high oxalate intake is a strong and independent risk factor for high urine oxalate, then one would expect vegetarians, whose oxalate intake may be expected to be quite high, to have a higher calcium oxalate stone incidence than nonvegetarians, and this is not the case. Other causes for high urine oxalate must be explored and ruled out before the reflexive recommendation to restrict oxalate.

- ***Oxalate restriction demonizes healthy foods and may compromise intake of stone inhibitors.*** Patients who peruse lists of high-oxalate foods, which largely consist of fruits and vegetables, frequently ask, "What can I eat?" and comment, "I thought I was supposed to eat fruits and vegetables." A general oxalate restriction, without isolating the very few foods with both a high oxalate content and high oxalate bioavailability, threatens the quality of patients' diets and encourages a negative association with some very healthy foods. Oxalate restriction may also interfere with or contradict recommendations patients have received for other aspects of their health, such as eating a high number of fruits and vegetables to prevent cancer or cardiovascular disease. Also, many of the foods highest in oxalate are also those highest in phytate (a potent inhibitor of calcium stones in urine), magnesium (an inhibitor of calcium oxalate stones), and fiber, which may be useful in regulating calcium absorption and in providing prebiotic material for the growth and colonization of healthy gut flora.

- *A focus on dietary oxalate restriction may minimize or even supplant other, more important clinical risk factors (e.g., high urinary calcium or uric acid, low urinary citrate or magnesium, acid urine, low volume).* Some patients, especially with multiple or complex risks, may require the introduction of one therapy at a time. Urinary calcium and other factors, such as volume, citrate, and magnesium, are important risk factors. Perhaps these could be more easily targeted and resolved with the desired effect of reduced calcium oxalate stone recurrence. Recently, some have challenged the notion that urine oxalate concentrations are more important than urine calcium concentrations with respect to calcium oxalate stone formation [61]. If true, then more attention on urinary calcium excretion, as opposed to urine oxalate concentration, is warranted.

- *We may be incorrectly diagnosing hyperoxaluria.* Data from well-designed studies have confirmed inter-laboratory variability in 24-h oxalate analysis [62]. If hyperoxaluria is diagnosed as a risk factor when it is not, a dietary oxalate restriction would have no value and may have any of the unwanted effects previously described. Even if the diagnosis from an individual 24-h urine collection is correct, categorizing a patient as "hyperoxaluric" on the basis of one collection may not be appropriate. The intake of oxalate is known to vary depending on the season and within a given time period [34, 35]. A one-time 24-h urine collection indicating high urine oxalate may not appropriately reflect a patient's true risk profile, especially if he/she had transient high urine oxalate from the intake of a food or beverage not typically consumed.

- *Dietary oxalate restriction requires a concomitant calcium restriction in order to maintain suitably low calcium oxalate supersaturation.* The restriction of calcium to below the recommended amount (1,000 mg per day for most adults) [16] could have unwanted health effects, particularly on bone health in those that are at risk for premature bone loss. Moreover, though underappreciated, there is evidence that lower oxalate intakes may increase urinary calcium excretion. Although not a primary outcome of the study, Penniston et al. noted that dietary oxalate was inversely correlated with urinary calcium excretion [63]. In this sense, oxalate is a calcium binder. Could dietary oxalate therefore have therapeutic benefit in regulating calcium absorption in those thought to have hyperabsorptive calciuria?

- *Food values vary: are we correctly restricting the truly high-oxalate foods?* There are different reported oxalate values for many foods and beverages. Inter-laboratory variability in measurements as well as the use of different testing procedures contributes to this problem. Also, other factors influence the oxalate content of foods; these include the maturity of the plant when harvested, soil and environmental conditions in the plant's growing location, and cooking and preparation procedures [64]. We may never be able to claim with certainty, for example, that a potato grown in the Midwest has the same oxalate content as one grown in the Northeast or that beans harvested and consumed in a less mature state have equivalent oxalate content as those left on the vine to mature longer. Given these problems, unnecessary restriction of some plant foods may go hand in hand with dietary oxalate restriction.

- ***The bioavailability of dietary oxalate is more important than the amount of oxalate consumed.*** It is now appreciated that potassium and sodium oxalate are well-absorbed sources of oxalate due to their solubility in chyme, the product of gastric digestion. Conversely, foods that have a predominance of calcium or magnesium oxalate would result in less oxalate absorbed due to the relative insolubility of these compounds. Restricting foods based only on their oxalate content may result in the unnecessary restriction of foods that would not be implicated in contributing to high urine oxalate. Without assessing oxalate bioavailability, a low oxalate diet based on the oxalate content of foods removes otherwise healthy foods from patients' diets.

- ***Dietary oxalate restriction restricts the diversity of gut flora and reduces the capacity to handle an occasional high oxalate load.*** Humans ideally have about 3 pounds of gut flora within their gastrointestinal tract. Gastrointestinal bacteria are known to exert wide-ranging health benefits. Recent studies confirm that both the composition and the amount of gut flora are directly influenced by diet [65, 66]. Oxalotrophic bacteria in the gastrointestinal tracts of humans and animals were reported first by Barner and Gallimore [67]. Oxalate degradation by microbes is recognized as an important means to regulate oxalate absorption [68, 69]. In ruminants, increased dietary oxalate induces the selection of oxalate-degrading bacteria and makes it possible for the host to tolerate quantities of oxalate that would otherwise be toxic or even lethal [70]. Oxalate restriction in humans may limit the colonization of oxalate-degrading bacteria, potentially leading to compromised degradation capacity when the occasional or even infrequent high-oxalate food or meal is consumed.

## Oxalate Absorption: A Better Clinical Target than Intake?

- ***Calcium intake regulates oxalate absorption.*** Oxalate is absorbed throughout the gastrointestinal tract, including stomach, small, and large intestines. Most absorption is thought to occur in the small intestine [71]. Typically, the amount of oxalate absorbed is much less than that consumed and is usually estimated at 5–10 % of total oxalate intake [72, 73]. Controlling oxalate absorption may make a more appropriate clinical focus, as it is widely known that calcium intake is inversely associated with calcium oxalate stones and urinary oxalate excretion. While distributed calcium intake at meals, presumably timed to match the intake of oxalate [74] has been recommended, recent data show that simply having adequate calcium "on board," regardless of its timing may be effective [75]. The use of calcium supplements should be reserved for those with severe malabsorption and whose dietary calcium intake, for whatever reason(s), is incapable of being normalized.

- ***Magnesium may be underutilized as an oxalate binder.*** Some data show a favorable effect of magnesium supplementation in the reduction of urinary oxalate excretion [76], especially when consumed at the same time as an oral oxalate load [77]. Magnesium is capable of binding with oxalate both in the gut, reducing oxalate absorption, and also in urine, enhancing the solubility of oxalate. But a review on the topic revealed that the efficacy of magnesium supplementation as an oxalate binder may be less than optimal, particularly if implemented as monotherapy [78]. Further research is warranted, especially in carefully selected subjects whose urinary oxalate excretion is thought to be driven largely by excessive oxalate absorption as magnesium supplementation in those whose urinary oxalate is largely from biosynthesis, for example, would not be expected to benefit.

- ***Probiotics and/or probiotic-rich foods and beverages could be stressed as a way to reduce oxalate absorption.*** This strategy, in addition to directly affecting oxalate absorption, may have additional health benefits. The question of why studies to date have yielded mixed results was recently discussed [79]. As suggested previously, the lack of observed effect may be due to inappropriate subject selection. In other words, to test whether gut bacteria reduce oxalate absorption by degrading oxalate, it is reasonable to assume that a positive effect would be observed only if low oxalate-degrading potential was the suspected problem. The "dilution" of studies with subjects who have variable causes for their hyperoxaluria may have thus contributed to the unclear body of results. Little attention has been placed on the dietary consumption of prebiotics, diet-derived constituents that feed and promote the growth of oxalate-degrading bacteria. A study in dogs and cats examined the effect of different food-derived prebiotics (fructooligosaccharides, guar gum, inulin, lactitol, gum Arabic, and maltodextrin) on gastrointestinal bacterial profile [80]. Results indicated that manipulation of the diet for these prebiotics could enhance oxalate degradation, resulting in reduced oxalate excreted in urine. As noted in the previous section, reduced dietary intake of prebiotic material promoting oxalate-degrading bacteria could diminish the oxalate degradation potential in the gut.

- ***Low fat diets may reduce calcium saponification and therefore be useful in reducing oxalate absorption.*** While the diets of some stone formers may be balanced with respect to overall macronutrient composition, others may have a high fat intake. Currently, total fat is recommended to be less than 30 % of total calories; some advise an upper intake of 20 %. The fat intake of many Americans exceeds this. Dietary fat intake by calcium oxalate stone formers is not a major clinical target currently. But data suggest that patients with suspected malabsorption may benefit from reduced fat intake as a positive linear relationship between urinary oxalate and fecal fat in patients was observed [81]. This makes sense as fatty acids are known to complex with calcium in the gastrointestinal tract to form calcium "soaps"[82]. Thus, by reducing dietary fat, more calcium is theoretically available to bind oxalate.

  Naya et al. [83] found that the intake of animal fat, which can contribute a large component of saturated and polyunsaturated fats, was associated with urinary oxalate excretion. The same group also found dietary arachidonic acid (a polyunsaturated omega-6 fatty acid found primarily in animal foods) to be associated with increased urinary oxalate [84]. Others, however, have not found such an association [85]. While more research is needed, another potential benefit of reducing the fat intake of calcium oxalate stone formers would be that overall caloric intake is reduced, potentially leading to weight loss. While weight loss per se has not been studied with respect to calcium oxalate stone recurrence, body mass is positively associated with kidney stone risk [86, 87]. Questions as to the efficacy of this approach, as well as to whether all fats are equal with respect to their calcium-saponifying potential, would need to be addressed before general promotion as a preventive strategy.

- ***Controlling malabsorption, if contributing to high urine oxalate, may require strategies not necessarily associated with reducing stone risk.*** Individuals with short bowel syndrome or other bowel conditions resulting in malabsorption are prone to calcium oxalate urolithiasis [33]. There are many accepted clinical nutrition strategies to manage malabsorption and diarrhea that may be useful in the setting of stone prevention. The goals of these measures typically include those aimed at increasing or slowing gut transit time, reducing gastric hypersecretion, and maintaining optimal gut bacteria concentrations. Tools used to achieve these goals include administration of pancreatic enzymes or bile acid binders; manipulation of dietary fiber, carbohydrates, and fat; and supplementation with probiotics, medium-chain triglycerides, and/or fiber. In patients whose malabsorption is suspected as the primary cause of their stones, prevention may be achieved by use of these methods, in concert with clinical nutrition consultation.

## Oxalate Biosynthesis: Are Dietary Factors Relevant?

- ***The extent to which oxalate biosynthesis can be reduced in the idiopathic calcium oxalate stone former by limiting precursors is debated.*** Dietary factors associated with increased oxalate production include oxalate precursors, such as ascorbate [88, 89], glycine, glycolate [90], and hydroxyproline [91]. Fructose, by unknown mechanisms, is also theorized as a promoter of oxalate synthesis [92, 93]. While it may seem appealing to recommend reduced intake of these dietary factors, problems arise when patients believe that food sources of ascorbic acid (vitamin C) must be reduced. While high intakes of vitamin C supplements >1,000 mg/d are associated with higher urinary oxalate [28, 94, 95], there are no data to suggest that the intake of fruits and vegetables rich in vitamin C cause increased oxalate biosynthesis. Restriction of these foods could compromise patients' overall intake of fruits and vegetables, which may have been recommended to elicit other favorable effects (e.g., reducing dietary acid load or increasing urinary stone inhibitors).

While fructose is associated in some studies with higher urinary oxalate [28, 93], attempts to confirm this in humans have been unsuccessful [96]. Fructose is available in the diet either from sucrose (glucose + fructose) or high fructose corn syrup. Consumption, especially from corn syrup, has increased exponentially over the past 40 years [97] and is implicated in increasing obesity rates [98]. Fructose comprises as much or more than half the total carbohydrate content of many fruits. Indeed, fruits are a major contributor to fructose in the diet [99]. As with recommendations to limit ascorbate intake, patients may be confused about how to limit fructose intake without limiting fruits. Care should be taken that patients understand that fructose from whole fruits is not harmful, even if several servings are consumed daily. If a limited fructose regimen is advised, sources such as high-sugar beverages, items sweetened with high fructose corn syrup, and highly processed carbohydrate foods should be the target.

Other food-derived precursors for oxalate synthesis are proposed to come from meats and other animal-derived foods, such as gelatin. While dietary patterns rich in "animal protein" have been long associated with increased calcium oxalate stone risk, the influence specifically of flesh and flesh-derived products on urinary oxalate excretion has only been recently studied. Nguyen et al. observed higher urinary oxalate excretion in some idiopathic calcium oxalate stone formers while on a high-meat protein diet. The authors theorized that a subset of stone formers may be "sensitive" to meat protein [100]. Knight et al. contradicted this finding in a similar feeding study, but subjects were not stone formers [101]. The flesh of both land- and marine-habited animals is rich in nonessential amino acids, some of which are direct precursors to oxalate biosynthesis. Knight et al. provided gelatin, an animal-derived product rich in hydroxyproline, to humans and observed increased urinary oxalate excretion [102], presumably from the metabolism of hydroxyproline to glyoxylate, an immediate oxalate precursor.

- ***The extent to which oxalate biosynthesis can be reduced in the idiopathic calcium oxalate stone former by increasing inhibitors is debated.*** Dietary factors suggested to reduce oxalate production include pyridoxine and fish oil. Pyridoxine (vitamin $B_6$) in high dosages may be effective in some patients with PH1 as it is a cofactor for an enzyme that prevents oxalate synthesis. Whether pyridoxine (vitamin $B_6$) supplementation is effective in patients with idiopathic hyperoxaluria is debated. There is a role for vitamin $B_6$ repletion in patients who are deficient [49], but vitamin $B_6$ deficiency is uncommon in the USA. What about patients who are already replete for this vitamin? Is supplementation useful in reducing oxalate synthesis? Epidemiologic studies suggest that supplemental vitamin $B_6$ intake is inversely associated with symptomatic kidney stones in women [103] but not in men [104]. Yet, the concentration of vitamin $B_6$ metabolites in idiopathic calcium oxalate stone formers does not appear different from non-stone formers [105]. While some data are supportive for pyridoxine supplementation along with other nutrition recommendations [50, 106] or in conjunction with supplemental magnesium [107], others are not [108]. There appears to be no consensus on the dosage of supplementation necessary to achieve maximal effect.

In controlled interventions, omega-3 fatty acids have been studied for their potential to reduce urinary oxalate excretion [47, 48, 109, 110]. Dietary omega-3 fatty acids are alpha-linolenic acid (ALA), DHA, and EPA. DHA and EPA are available from cold water fish and as over-the-counter supplements (e.g., fish oil), whereas ALA is from plant sources. Results of these studies have shown reductions in urinary oxalate. Siener et al. [47] propose that the effect may not be on oxalate biosynthesis but, rather, on oxalate transport, which appears to be reduced with omega-3 fatty acid supplementation via cell membrane changes in fatty acid composition. Future work is needed to identify dosages, long-term safety, and whether the therapy is useful in all patients with high urine oxalate or a specific subset thereof.

## Calcium Oxalate Supersaturation: A More Effective Therapeutic Target than 24-H Urine Oxalate Concentration?

- ***Urine calcium may actually be equal to oxalate in its contribution to calcium oxalate stone formation*** [61]. Thus, arduous control of urinary oxalate excretion may be misplaced. In those with intransigent high urine oxalate, or with mild hyperoxaluria, a shift toward urinary calcium excretion as the major risk factor to be treated may yield greater benefit.
- ***Urinary inhibitors of calcium oxalate stones should receive greater attention as clinical targets against calcium oxalate stone formation.*** Nutrition therapy is sometimes overly associated with the restriction of certain foods and beverages or with recommendations about what *not* to eat. Many have argued that a more positive focus (i.e., on the foods and beverages patients *can* eat) would improve compliance, adherence, and clinical results. Greater attention to increasing urinary stone inhibitors, as opposed to restricting oxalate, may be warranted. Magnesium oxalate (glushinskite) is a more soluble complex in urine than calcium oxalate. As early as 1929, a low magnesium intake was associated with high urinary oxalate excretion [111]. Efforts to increase dietary magnesium intake, either from foods or a combination of foods and supplements, may result in reduced calcium oxalate supersaturation in urine without the need to alter urinary oxalate excretion.

Phytate (myo-inositol hexaphosphate) is a little-known inhibitor of calcium stones as it binds with calcium to form a soluble complex in urine. Its urinary excretion can be manipulated in humans with diet [112]. As there are other health benefits associated with high-phytate diets, including prevention of cancer and cardiovascular calcification, recommendations to increase phytate from foods could be provided. There may be controversy about this, however, as most of the high-phytate foods are also those highest in oxalate; these include nuts, whole cereals, and some legumes. Unfortunately, commercial laboratories do not currently measure urinary phytate excretion. The impact of increased urinary phytate on the calcium oxalate stone formation risk would be difficult to ascertain.

Citrate forms a soluble complex with calcium. Potassium citrate has long been used in medical management to increase urinary citrate excretion. Citrate salts, albeit in lower doses than prescribed pharmacologically, are also consumed in the diet. Much of the potassium obtained from fruits and vegetables, for example, is complexed with citrate. Citrate, whether from potassium or some other citrate salt, is metabolized in the liver to bicarbonate, and this confers an alkaline load to the kidneys, allowing for increased citraturia. Urinary citrate excretion may be appreciably increased, thereby reducing calcium oxalate stone formation risk, by consuming 5 or more fruits and vegetables daily [113]. Dietary citric acid, an organic acid found in many fruits and vegetables and also used as a flavoring agent, is the protonated form of citrate. Its intake was not previously thought to influence urinary citrate excretion as its conversion to bicarbonate in the liver leaves a free $H^+$ ion, resulting in a net neutral effect on renal acid-base balance with questionable capacity to influence renal citrate excretion. Yet recent studies predict a citraturic effect from citric and other organic acids [114–116], and these could play a role in the reduction of calcium oxalate stone formation risk without having to impose a dietary restriction of high-oxalate foods.

## Discussion

Oxalic acid in many forms abounds in nature and plays a useful role in plants as well as in some human activities. There is a potential role for oxalate in attenuating the effects of rising atmospheric carbon dioxide concentration via the microbial degradation of oxalate in soil. Urinary oxalate excretion, however, is a concern for calcium oxalate stone formation in humans and animalia of all types. Oxalate originates from both exogenous (diet, supplements) and endogenous sources. Although there is wide variability between individuals, a 50 % contribution to urinary oxalate is estimated from each source. Oxalate is not a nutrient and is neither regulated nor used by humans; therefore, exogenous oxalate that is absorbed in the gastrointestinal tract must be excreted. Excretion is also the only route for elimination of the oxalate produced in vivo by metabolism (biosynthesis). There is no pharmacologic agent designed specifically to reduce urine oxalate. Reduction or maintenance of the amount of oxalate that is both absorbed and synthesized is therefore the main objective of medical management to prevent calcium oxalate stone formation.

Except in the case of the primary hyperoxalurias, in which case a genetic defect can be identified, hyperoxaluria is multifactorial. Its contributors include:

- Intake of oxalate and oxalate precursors
- Gastrointestinal handling of oxalate and gastrointestinal health in general
- Bile acid metabolism
- Intake of minerals that prevent oxalate absorption
- Intake of fat and other diet-derived constituents that favor oxalate absorption
- The relative presence of oxalotrophic bacteria in the gastrointestinal tract
- Underlying medical conditions that lead to alterations in any of the above

As with other medical conditions, the etiology of the derangement informs the therapy. In the case of high urine oxalate, determining the primary contributor(s) is not always straightforward, as there may not always be reliable measures to substantiate the putative cause and as individuals vary greatly with respect to the factors that contribute to oxalate excretion. This has led to the implementation of therapies that may not be aimed at the correct problem and to the layering on of multiple strategies with the hope that one of them will accomplish the desired effect. In addition to problems associated with differential individual responses to therapy, effects of the various medical management strategies on high urine oxalate have not been critically evaluated either alone or in concert. This has resulted in a lack of evidence to drive clinical standards of care, leading to differential practice patterns and results, data from which are difficult to interpret and assess. Finally, mechanisms of action for many of the strategies either in use or under consideration are not known. Given these problems, it is not surprising that there are controversies in the medical management of high urine oxalate and calcium oxalates stone formers.

## Conclusion

Oxalate has been controversial in calcium oxalate stone formers, partly due to a lack of complete understanding of the disease process. Although hyperoxaluria can frequently be managed effectively by calcium supplementation and/or calcium intake timed with meals, it is less clear how valuable dietary oxalate restriction can be in stone formers. Moreover, treatments, such as probiotics, inhibitors such as vitamin $B_6$, omega-3 fatty acids, and limitation of precursor intake (e.g., ascorbic acid) remain largely unproven. Most notably, hyperoxaluria can be quite severe, especially associated with bowel disorders, including gastric bypass. The difficult paradigm presented by this population alone validates the need for more answers.

## References


1. Aliano NP, Ellis MD. Oxalic acid: a prospective tool for reducing Varroa mite populations in package bees. Exp Appl Acarol 2009;48:303–9.
2. Gillam DG, Coventry JF, Manning RH, Newman HN, Bulman JS. Comparison of two desensitizing agents for the treatment of cervical dentine sensitivity. Endod Dent Traumatol. 1997;13:36–9.
3. Lazzarini L, Salvadori O. A reassessment of the formation of the patina called scialbatura. Stud Conser. 1989;34:20–6.
4. Russ J, Loyd DH, Boutton TW. A paleoclimate reconstruction for southwestern Texas using oxalate residue from lichen as a paleoclimate proxy. Quart Int. 2000;67:29–36.
5. Caliskan M. The metabolism of oxalate. Turk J Zool. 2000;24:103–6.
6. Franceschi VR, Nakata PA. Calcium oxalate in plants: formation and function. Ann Rev Plant Biol. 2005;56:41–71.
7. Cailleau G, Braissant O, Verrecchia EP. Turning sunlight into stone: the oxalate-carbonate pathway in a tropical tree system. Biogeosciences. 2011;8:1755–67.
8. Beazley MJ, Rickman RD, Ingram DK, Boutton TW, Russ J. Natural abundances of carbon isotopes ($^{14}C$, $^{13}C$) in lichens and calcium oxalate pruina: implications for archaeological and paleoenvironmental studies. Radiocarbon. 2002;44:675–83.

9. Freeman BC, Beattie GA. 2008. An overview of plant defenses against pathogens and herbivores. The Plant Health Instructor. doi:10.1094/PHI-I-2008-0226-01.
10. Monje PV, Baran EJ. Characterization of calcium oxalates generated as biominerals in cacti. Plant Physiol. 2002;128:707–13.
11. Ma JF, Hiradate S, Matsumoto H. High aluminum resistance in buckwheat. Plant Physiol. 1998;117:753–9.
12. Mithril C, Dragsted. LO. Safety evaluation of some wild plants in the New Nordic diet. Food Chem Toxicol. 2012;50:4461–7.
13. Harvard School of Public Health Nutrition Department's file. 2013. https://regepi.bwh.harvard.edu/health/Oxalate/files. Accessed 7 Aug 2013.
14. Cartery C, Faquer S, Karras A, Cointault O, Buscail L, Modesto A, et al. Oxalate nephropathy associated with chronic pancreatitis. Clin J Am Soc Nephrol. 2011;6:1895–902.
15. Fishbein GA, Micheletti RG, Currier JS, Singer E, Fishbein MC. Atherosclerotic oxalosis in coronary arteries. Cardiovasc Pathol. 2008;17:117–23.
16. Institute of Medicine (US) Committee to Review Dietary Reference Intakes for Vitamin D and Calcium. P. 2. Overview of Calcium. In: Ross AC, Taylor CL, Yaktine AL, et al., editors. Dietary reference intakes for calcium and vitamin D. Washington, DC: National Academies Press (US); 2011. http://www.ncbi.nlm.nih.gov/books/NBK56060/. Accessed 8 Aug 2013.
17. Knapp EL. Factors influencing the urinary excretion of calcium in normal persons. J Clin Invest. 1947;26:182–202.
18. Trinchieri A. Diet and renal stone formation. Minerva Med. 2013;104:41–54.
19. Dunlop JC. The excretion of oxalate acid in urine, and its bearing on the pathological condition known as oxaluria. J Pathol Bacteriol. 1896;3:389–429.
20. Holmes RP, Goodman HO, Assimos DG. Contribution of dietary oxalate to urinary oxalate excretion. Kidney Int. 2001;59:270–6.
21. Freel RW, Hatch M, Green M, Soleimani M. Ileal oxalate absorption and urinary oxalate excretion are enhanced in Slc26a6 null mice. Am J Physiol Gastrointest Liver Physiol. 2006;290:19–28.
22. Liu RH. Dietary bioactive compounds and their health implications. J Food Sci. 2013;78:A18–25.
23. Martino HS, Martin BR, Weaver CM, Bressan J, Esteves EA, Costa NM. Zinc and iron bioavailability of genetically modified soybeans in rats. J Food Sci. 2007;72:689–95.
24. Baldwin H. An experimental study of oxaluria, with special reference to its fermentive origin. J Exp Med. 1900;5:27–46.
25. Shah J, Whitfield HN. Urolithiasis through the ages. BJU Int. 2002;89:801–10.
26. Robijn S, Hoppe B, Vervaet BA, D'Haese PC, Verhulst A. Hyperoxaluria: a gut-kidney axis? Kidney Int. 2011;80:1146–58.
27. Holmes RP, Kennedy M. Estimation of the oxalate content of foods and daily oxalate intake. Kidney Int. 2000;57:1662–7.
28. Taylor EN, Curhan GC. Determinants of 24-hour urinary oxalate excretion. Clin J Am Soc Nephrol. 2008;3:1453–60.
29. Hallson PC, Rose GA. Crystalluria in normal subjects and in stone formers with and without thiazide and cellulose phosphate treatment. Br J Urol. 1976;48:515–24.
30. Lopez M, Hoppe B. History, epidemiology and regional diversities of urolithiasis. Pedatr Nephrol. 2010;25:49–59.
31. Curhan GC, Willett WC, Speizer FE, Stampfer MJ. Twenty-four-hour urine chemistries and the risk of kidney stones among women and men. Kidney Int. 2001;59:2290–8.
32. Curhan GC, Taylor EN. 24-h uric acid excretion and the risk of kidney stones. Kidney Int. 2008;73:489–96.
33. Worcester EM. Stones from bowel disease. Endocrinol Metab Clin North Am. 2002;31:979–99.
34. Juuti M, Heinonen OP, Alhava EM. Seasonal variation in urinary excretion of calcium, oxalate, magnesium and phosphate on free and standard mineral diet in men with urolithasis. Scand J Urol Nephrol. 1981;15:137–41.

35. Robertson WG, Peacock M, Marshall RW, Speed R, Nordin BE. Seasonal variations in the composition of urine in relation to calcium stone-formation. Clin Sci Mol Med. 1975;49:597–602.
36. Finlayson B. Physiochemical aspects of urolithiasis. Kidney Int. 1978;13:344–60.
37. Robertson WG, Peacock M, Heyburn PJ, Marshall DH, Clark PB. Risk factors in calcium stone disease of the urinary tract. Br J Urol. 1978;50:449–54.
38. Robertson WG, Peacock M. The cause of idiopathic calcium stone disease: hypercalciuria or hyperoxaluria? Nephron. 1980;26:105–10.
39. Rodgers A. Aspects of calcium oxalate crystallization: theory, in vitro studies, and in vivo implementation. J Am Soc Nephrol. 1999;10:S351–4.
40. Caspary WF, Tonissen J, Lankisch PG. 'Enteral' hyperoxaluria. Effect of cholestyramine, calcium, neomycin, and bile acids on intestinal oxalate absorption in man. Acta Hepatogastroenterol (Stuttg). 1977;24:193–200.
41. Smith LH, Fromm H, Hofmann AF. Acquired hyperoxaluria, nephrolithiasis, and intestinal disease. Description of a syndrome. N Engl J Med. 1972;286:1371–5.
42. Nordenvall B, Backman L, Larsson L, Tiselius HG. Effects of calcium, aluminum, magnesium and cholestyramine on hyperoxaluria in patients with jejunoileal bypass. Acta Chir Scand. 1983;149:93–8.
43. Emmett M, Guirl MJ, Santa Ana CA, Porter JL, Neimark S, Hofmann AF, et al. Conjugated bile acid replacement therapy reduces urinary oxalate excretion in short bowel syndrome. Am J Kidney Dis. 2003;41:230–7.
44. Siener R, Petzold J, Bitterlich N, Alteheld B. Metzner C. Determinants of urolithiasis in patients with intestinal fat malabsorption. Urology. 2013;81:17–24.
45. Rankin AC, Walsh SB, Summers SA, Owen MP, Mansell MA. Acute oxalate nephropathy causing late renal transplant dysfunction due to enteric hyperoxaluria. Am J Transplant. 2008;8:1755–8.
46. Miyaoka R, Monga M. Use of traditional Chinese medicine in the management of urinary stone disease. Int Braz J Urol. 2009;35:396–405.
47. Siener R, Jansen B, Watzer B, Hesse A. Effect of n-3 fatty acid supplementation on urinary risk factors for calcium oxalate stone formation. J Urol. 2011;185:719–24.
48. Lange J, Mufarrij P, Easter L, Knight J, Holmes R, Assimos D. The impact of fish oil supplementation on endogenous oxalate synthesis and urinary oxalate excretion. J Urol. 2013;189:e925.
49. Mydlik M, Derzsiova K. Vitamin $B_6$ and oxalaic acid in clinical nephropathy. J Ren Nutr. 2010;20:S95–102.
50. Ortiz-Alvarado O, Miyaoka R, Kriedberg C, Moeding A, Stessman M, Monga M. Pyridoxine and dietary counseling for the management of idiopathic hyperoxaluria in stone-forming patients. Urology. 2011;77:1054–8.
51. Dahiya T, Pundir CS. In vivo oxalate degradation by liposome encapsulated oxalate oxidase in rat model of hyperoxaluria. Indian J Med Res. 2013;137:136–41.
52. Sahin N. Oxalotrophic bacteria. Res Microbiol. 2003;154:399–407.
53. Liebman M, Al-Wahsh IA. Probiotics and other key determinants of dietary oxalate absorption. Adv Nutr. 2011;2:254–60.
54. Abratt VR, Reid SJ. Oxalate-degrading bacteria of the human gut as probiotics in the management of kidney stone disease. Adv Appl Microbiol. 2010;72:63–87.
55. Lieske JC, Goldfarb DS, De Simone C, Regnier C. Use of a probiotic to decrease enteric hyperoxaluria. Kidney Int. 2005;68:1244–9.
56. Fink HA, Akornor JW, Garimella PS, MacDonald R, Cutting A, Rutks IR, et al. Diet, fluid, or supplements for secondary prevention of nephrolithiasis: a systematic review and meta-analysis of randomized trials. Eur Urol. 2009;56:72–80.
57. Lieske JC, Tremaine WJ, De Simone C, O'Connor HM, Li X, Bergstralh EJ, et al. Diet, but not oral probiotics, effectively reduces urinary oxalate excretion and calcium oxalate supersaturation. Kidney Int. 2010;78:1178–85.

58. Pang R, Linnes MP, O'Connor HM, Li X, Bergstralh E, Lieske JC. Controlled metabolic diet reduces calcium oxalate supersaturation but not oxalate excretion after bariatric surgery. Urology. 2012;80:250–4.
59. Taylor EN, Curhan GC. Oxalate intake and the risk for nephrolithiasis. J Am Soc Nephrol. 2007;18:2198–204.
60. Penniston KL, Wojciechowski KF, Nakada SY. Dietary oxalate: what's important and what isn't for patients with calcium oxalate stones? J Urol. 2011;185:e824–5.
61. Pak CY, Adams-Huet B, Poindexter JR, Pearle MS, Peterson RD, Moe OW. Rapid communication: relative effect of urinary calcium and oxalate on saturation of calcium oxalate. Kidney Int. 2004;66:2032–7.
62. Maalouf NM, Adams Huet B, Pasch A, Lieske JC, Asplin JR, Siener R, et al. Variability in urinary oxalate measurements between six international laboratories. Nephrol Dial Transplant. 2011;26:3954–9.
63. Penniston KL, Jones AN, Nakada SY, Hansen KE. Vitamin D repletion does not alter urinary calcium excretion in healthy postmenopausal women. BJU Int. 2009;104:1512–6.
64. Massey LK. Food oxalate: factors affecting measurement, biological variation, and bioavailability. J Am Diet Assoc. 2007;107:1191–4.
65. Wu GD, Chen J, Hoffmann C, Bittinger K, Chen YY, Keilbaugh SA, et al. Linking long-term dietary patterns with gut microbial enterotypes. Science. 2011;334:105–8.
66. Flint HJ. The impact of nutrition on the human microbiome. Nutr Rev. 2012;70:S10–3.
67. Barner HH, Gallimore EJ. The metabolism of oxalic acid in the animal body. Biochem J. 1940;34:144–8.
68. Talapatra SK, Ray SC, Sen KC. Calcium assimilation in ruminants on oxalate-rich diet. J Agri Sci. 1948;38:163–73.
69. Morris MP, Garcia-Rivera J. The destruction of oxalate by rumen contents of cows. J Dairy Sci. 1955;38:1169.
70. Allison MJ, Cook HM. Oxalate degradation by microbes of the large bowel of herbivores: the effect of dietary oxalate. Science. 1981;212:675–6.
71. Knauf F, Ko N, Jiang Z, Robertson WG, Van Itallie CM, Anderson JM, et al. Net intestinal transport of oxalate reflects passive absorption and SLC26A6-mediated secretion. J Am Soc Nephrol. 2011;22:2247–55.
72. Knight J, Jiang J, Wood KD, Holmes RP, Assimos DG. Oxalate and sucralose absorption in idiopathic calcium oxalate stone formers. Urology. 2011;78:e9–13.
73. Voss S, Hesse A, Zimmerman DJ, Sauerbruch T, von Unruh GE. Intestinal oxalate absorption is higher in idiopathic calcium oxalate stone formers than in healthy controls: measurements with the [(13)C2] oxalate absorption test. J Urol. 2006;175:1711–5.
74. Penniston KL, Nakada SY. Effect of dietary changes on urinary oxalate excretion and calcium oxalate supersaturation in patients with hyperoxaluric stone formation. Urology. 2009;73:484–9.
75. Lange JN, Wood KD, Mufarrij PW, Callahan MF, Easter L, Knight J, et al. The impact of dietary calcium and oxalate ratios on stone risk. Urology. 2012;79:1226–9.
76. Voss S, Zimmerman DJ, Hesse A, von Unruh GE. The effect of oral administration of calcium and magnesium on intestinal oxalate absorption in humans. Isotopes Environ Health Stud. 2004;40:199–205.
77. Zimmerman DJ, Voss S, von Unruh GE, Hesse A. Importance of magnesium in absorption and excretion of oxalate. Urol Int. 2005;74:262–7.
78. Massey L. Magnesium therapy for nephrolithiasis. Magnes Res. 2005;18:123–6.
79. Borghi L, Nouvenne A, Meschi T. Probiotics and dietary manipulations in calcium oxalate nephrolithiasis: two sides of the same coin? Kidney Int. 2010;78:1063–5.
80. Weese JS, Weese HE, Yuricek L, Rousseau J. Oxalate degradation by intestinal lactic acid bacteria in dogs and cats. Vet Microbiol. 2004;101:161–6.
81. Rampton DS, Kasidas GP, Rose GA, Sarner M. Oxalate loading test: a screening test for steatorrhoea. Gut. 1979;20:1089–94.

82. Steiner MS, Morton RA. Nutritional and gastrointestinal complications of the use of bowel segments in the lower urinary tract. Urol Clin North Am. 1991;18:743–54.

83. Naya Y, Ito H, Masai M, Yamaguchi K. Effect of dietary intake on urinary oxalate excretion in calcium oxalate stone formers in their forties. Eur Urol. 2000;37:140–4.

84. Naya Y, Ito H, Masaai M, Yamaguchi K. Association of dietary fatty acids with urinary oxalate excretion in calcium oxalate stone-formers in their fourth decade. BJU Int. 2002;89:842–6.

85. Bailly GG, Norman RW, Thompson C. Effects of dietary fat on the urinary risk factors of calcium stone disease. Urology. 2000;56:40–4.

86. Taylor EN, Curhan GC. Body size and 24-hour urine composition. Am J Kidney Dis. 2006;48:905–15.

87. Eisner BH, Eisenberg ML, Stoller ML. Relationship between body mass index and quantitative 24-hour urine chemistries in patients with nephrolithiasis. Urology. 2010;75:1289–93.

88. Baxmann AC, De O G Mendonca C, Heilberg IP. Effect of vitamin C supplements on urinary oxalate and pH in calcium stone-forming patients. Kidney Int. 2003;63:1066–71.

89. Massey LK, Liebman M, Kynast-Gales SA. Ascorbate increases human oxaluria and kidney stone risk. J Nutr. 2005;135:1673–7.

90. Harris KS, Richardson KE. Glycolate in the diet and its conversion to urinary oxalate in the rat. Invest Urol. 1980;18:106–9.

91. Ribaya JD, Gershoff SN. Factors affecting endogenous oxalate synthesis and its excretion in feces and urine in rats. J Nutr. 1982;112:2161–9.

92. Taylor EN, Curhan GC. Fructose consumption and the risk of kidney stones. Kidney Int. 2008;73:207–12.

93. Nguyen NU, Dumoulin G, Henriet MT, Regnard J. Increase in urinary calcium and oxalate after fructose infusion. Horm Metab Res. 1995;27:155–8.

94. Traxer O, Huet B, Poindexter J, Pak CY, Pearle MS. Effect of ascorbic acid consumption on urinary stone risk factors. J Urol. 2003;170:397–401.

95. Thomas LD, Elinder CG, Tiselius HG, Wolk A, Akesson A. Ascorbic acid supplements and kidney stone incidence among men: a prospective study. JAMA Intern Med. 2013;173:386–8.

96. Knight J, Assimos DG, Easter L, Holmes RP. Metabolism of fructose to oxalate and glycolate. Horm Metab Res. 2010;42:868–73.

97. Bray GA. Energy and fructose from beverages sweetened with sugar or high-fructose corn syrup pose a health risk for some people. Adv Nutr. 2013;4:220–5.

98. Eilliott SS, Keim NL, Stern JS, Teff K, Havel PJ. Fructose, weight gain, and the insulin resistance syndrome. Am J Clin Nutr. 2002;76:911–22.

99. Marriott BP, Cole N, Lee E. National estimates of dietary fructose intake increased from 1977–2004 in the United States. J Nutr. 2009;139:1228S–35S.

100. Nguyen QV, Kalin A, Drouve U, Casez JP, Jaeger P. Sensitivity to meat protein intake and hyperoxaluria in idiopathic calcium stone formers. Kidney Int. 2001;59:2273–81.

101. Knight J, Jiang J, Assimos DG, Holmes RP. Hydroxyproline ingestion and urinary oxalate and glycolate excretion. Kidney Int. 2006;70:1929–34.

102. Knight J, Easter LH, Neiberg R, Assimos DG, Holmes RP. Increased protein intake on controlled oxalate diets does not increase urinary oxalate excretion. Urol Res. 2009;37:63–8.

103. Curhan GC, Willett WC, Speizer FE, Stampfer MJ. Intake of vitamins $B_6$ and C and the risk of kidney stones in women. J Am Soc Nephrol. 1999;10:840–5.

104. Curhan GC, Willett WC, Rimm EB, Stampfer MJ. A prospective study of the intake of vitamins C and $B_6$, and the risk of kidney stones in men. J Urol. 1996;155:1847–51.

105. Kaelin A, Casez JP, Jaeger P. Vitamin $B_6$ metabolites in idiopathic calcium stone formers: no evidence for a link to hyperoxaluria. Urol Res. 2004;32:61–8.

106. Rao TV, Choudhary VK. Effect of pyridoxine (vitamin $B_6$) supplementation on calciuria and oxaluria levels of some normal healthy persons and urinary stone patients. Indian J Clin Biochem. 2005;20:166–9.

107. Rattan V, Sidhu H, Vaidyanathan S, Thind SK, Nath R. Effect of combined supplementation of magnesium oxide and pyridoxine in calcium-oxalate stone formers. Urol Res. 1994;22:161–5.
108. Edwards P, Nemat S, Rose GA. Effects of oral pyridoxine upon plasma and 24-hour urinary oxalate levels in normal subjects and stone forms with idiopathic hypercalciuria. Urol Res. 1990;18:393–6.
109. Siener R, Alteheld B, Terjung B, Junghans B, Bitterlich N, Stehle P, et al. Change in the fatty acid pattern of erythrocyte membrane phospholipids after oral supplementation of specific fatty acids in patients with gastrointestinal diseases. Eur J Clin Nutr. 2010;64:410–8.
110. Buck AC, Davied RL, Harrison T. The protective role of eicosapentaenoic acid (EPA) in the pathogenesis of nephrolithiasis. J Urol. 1991;146:188–94.
111. Hammarsten G. Dietetic therapy in the formation of calcium oxalate calculi in the urinary passage. Acta Physiol. 1938;80:165–75.
112. Prieto RM, Fiol M, Perello J, Estruch R, Ros E, Sanchis P, Grases F. Effects of Mediterranean diets with low and high proportions of phytate-rich foods on the urinary phytate excretion. Eur J Nutr. 2010;49:321–6.
113. Meschi T, Maggiore U, Fiaccadori E, Schianchi T, Bosi S, Adorni G, et al. The effect of fruits and vegetables on urinary stone risk factors. Kidney Int. 2002;66:2402–10.
114. Eisner BH, Asplin JR, Goldfarb DS, Ahmad A, Stoller ML. Citrate, malate and alkali content in commonly consumed diet sodas: implications for nephrolithiasis treatment. J Urol. 2010;183:2419–23.
115. Baia Lda C, Baxmann AC, Moreira SR, Holmes RP, Heilberg IP. Noncitrus alkaline fruit: a dietary alternative for the treatment of hypocitraturic stone formers. J Endourol. 2012;26:1221–6.
116. Aras B, Kalfazade N, Tuqcu V, Kemahli E, Ozbay B, Polat H, et al. Can lemon juice be an alternative to potassium citrate in the treatment of urinary calcium stones in patients with hypocitraturia? A prospective randomized study. Urol Res. 2008;36:313–7.

# Chapter 3
# Dietary Calcium and Prevention of Calcium Stones: More or Less?

Jodi Antonelli and Margaret S. Pearle

## Introduction

Kidney stone disease is an increasingly common condition in the US. The National Health and Nutrition Examination Survey (NHANES) II and III datasets showed that the lifetime risk of forming stones among US adults rose significantly from 3.2 % in 1976 to 5.2 % in 1994 [1]. This trend has also been reflected in the most recent NHANES dataset (2007–2010) with the prevalence of stones in US men and women now estimated at 8.8 % [2]. Kidney stones are particularly distressful in part because they have a high propensity to recur with a rate ranging from 26 to 53 % [3, 4]. As the prevalence of stone disease rises, the associated morbidity and attendant costs to individuals and the health care system mount. An estimate of the total annual expenditure for urolithiasis in the US was calculated to be $ 2.1 billion in 2000, which represented a 50 % increase from estimates in 1994 [5]. Medical and surgical treatments of stones comprise a large portion of these costs; however, indirect costs including lost wages from time away from work have been estimated to increase the annual expenditure for stone disease in the US to a total of $ 5.1 billion [6].

Prevention of stone disease is the key to breaking the cycle of recurrence, patient suffering, and mounting costs. Dietary modifications are an attractive means to prevent stone formation because they are generally well tolerated and inexpensive. Although urinary (calcium) Ca is thought to play an important role in stone formation since hypercalciuria comprises the most common metabolic abnormality identified in stone formers and approximately 70–80 % of stones contain Ca [7–9], the impact of dietary Ca on urinary Ca levels and risk of urinary stones remains controversial. Moreover, the effect of altering dietary Ca potentially impacts not only stone formation but also bone health. Herein we review the evidence regarding dietary Ca and its effects on urinary Ca and stone risk.

M. S. Pearle (✉) · J. Antonelli
Department of Urology, University of Texas Southwestern Medical Center,
5324 Harry Hines Blvd., J8.106, Dallas, TX 75390-9110, USA
e-mail: margaret.pearle@utsouthwestern.edu

M. S. Pearle, S. Y. Nakada (eds.), *Practical Controversies in Medical Management of Stone Disease,* DOI 10.1007/978-1-4614-9575-8_3,
© Springer Science+Business Media New York 2014

## Role of Calcium in Stone Formation

The most common component of urinary calculi is Ca, with over 70 % of all stones containing Ca, primarily in the form of Ca oxalate or Ca phosphate [9,10]. Elevated urine Ca, or hypercalciuria, is the most prevalent metabolic abnormality identified in patients with Ca stones, and it is diagnosed in 30–60 % of adults with urolithiasis [11]. One of the potential sequelae of higher urinary Ca excretion is the formation of insoluble Ca salts that act as nidi for stone formation.

Over 50 years ago Hodgkinson and Pyrah noted that Ca stone formers had higher urinary Ca levels than non-stone-forming "normal" subjects. Among non-stone-forming men, 90 % had a urine Ca less than 300 mg (7.5 mmol)/day, and 90 % of non-stone-forming women had a urine Ca less than 250 mg (6.25 mmol)/day [12]. Parks and Coe defined hypercalciuria as urinary Ca excretion exceeding 4 mg/kg/day or greater than 7 mmol/day in men and greater than 6 mmol/day in women [13]. By the strictest definition, hypercalciuria has been defined as urinary Ca>200 mg/day after 1 week of adhering to a 400 mg Ca, 100 mg sodium diet [14]. However, although hypercalciuria is defined by urinary Ca levels that exceed a particular cut-point, urinary Ca is a continuous variable that likely demonstrates a spectrum of effects over its range, rather than inducing adverse effects occurring only after the level exceeds a threshold.

Hypercalciuria arises out of dysregulation at any site where large fluxes of Ca are tightly controlled, including the intestine, bone, and kidney [9]. Historically, hypercalciuria has been divided into three distinct subtypes based on pathophysiologic derangements at these three sites: absorptive, resorptive, and renal, respectively [15]. However, although this classification system has provided a framework for understanding the mechanisms and treatment of hypercalciuria, it is likely that metabolic dysregulation of Ca cannot be simplistically isolated to a single organ system. Rather, hypercalciuria is likely the result of multiple, interrelated pathophysiologic derangements [8]. As such, utilization of a classification system for hypercalciuria, apart from distinguishing primary hyperparathyroidism from all other forms of hypercalciuria, has not been associated with superior therapeutic efficacy and is therefore not routinely implemented in clinical practice [16]. Consequently, the term "idiopathic hypercalciuria" is used to describe a syndrome of stone formation for which the exact pathophysiologic mechanism is unknown but which is thought to be associated with hypercalciuria [17]. Over half of adult Ca stone formers are given a diagnosis of idiopathic hypercalciuria [18], and this nomenclature suggests that hypercalciuria and stone formation comprise a multifactorial disease process that cannot be attributed to derangements at a single organ site.

## Urinary Calcium and Stone Risk

Data from large epidemiologic studies as well as from a randomized, controlled trial (RCT) support a correlation between higher urine Ca and increased stone risk. Curhan and colleagues analyzed a subgroup of men and women from three large cohort studies, including both subjects who did ($n=807$) and did not ($n=239$) form stones during the course of observation, for whom 24-h urine specimens were available. The three cohort studies comprised the Nurses' Health Study I (NHS I) consisting of 121,700 female registered nurses aged 30–55, the Nurses' Health Study II (NHS II) consisting of 116,671 female registered nurses aged 25–42, and the Health Professionals Follow-up Study (HPFS) consisting of 51,529 male health professionals aged 40–75 years. The subjects in these large cohort studies completed biennial questionnaires regarding various aspects of their health including whether or not they had ever been diagnosed with a kidney stone as well as their frequency of intake of particular foods. After adjusting for other confounding factors, mean urinary Ca excretion was higher in those reporting a first-time stone than in those without stones in NHS I ($p=0.01$), NHS II ($p=0.06$), and HPFS ($p<0.001$). Among women, hypercalciuria was the most common urinary abnormality, occurring significantly more frequently among incident stone formers than in controls in NHS II ($p=0.03$) but not NHS I ($p=0.26$). Among men the most common abnormalities were hyperoxaluria, hyperuricosuria, and hypercalciuria, with hypercalciuria occurring significantly more frequently among stone formers than in controls ($p=0.02$). Indeed, on multivariate analysis, the risk of incident stone formation increased with increasing urinary Ca in both women ($p<0.001$) and men ($p=0.005$), supporting a contributory role for hypercalciuria in stone formation [19].

Indirect evidence supporting a pathogenetic role for Ca in stone formation comes from the finding that medications that lower urinary Ca have been shown to reduce stone recurrence rates. Pearle and coworkers performed a meta-analysis of RCTs evaluating drug treatments for the secondary prevention of Ca stone disease. Among 14 RCTs with 20 treatment arms assessing six different drug therapies, eight RCTs analyzed the benefit hypocalciuric agents (thiazides or a thiazide-like medication, indapamide) in preventing stone recurrence in recurrent Ca stone formers. Interestingly, although only two of the included studies were limited specifically to hypercalciuric patients, six of the eight trials demonstrated a significantly lower stone recurrence rate in the treatment arm compared to the control arm. Of note, the two studies that did not show a difference between groups had a mean duration of follow-up of less than 2 years, which may have been insufficient to show a difference. Analysis of the eight thiazide/indapamide trials demonstrated a statistically significant reduction in mean stone recurrence rates with treatment compared to placebo/no treatment ($p=0.02$). Furthermore, among the six thiazide/indapamide trials with appropriately expressed data, meta-analysis revealed a 21.3 % risk reduction in stone recurrence rates with active treatment compared with placebo/no treatment (95 % confidence interval [CI] −29.2 to −13.4 %; $p<0.001$) [20].

Escribano performed a Cochrane-based systematic review and meta-analysis of RCTs or quasi-RCTs that compared pharmacologic intervention to placebo in patients with idiopathic hypercalciuria treated for a minimum of four months with a follow-up of at least six months. Among these studies, four involved the use of thiazides or indapamide. They found a significant decrease in the number of stone recurrences in those treated with thiazides compared to the control group (relative risk (RR) 1.61, 95 % CI 1.33–1.96). Additionally the rate of stone formation expressed as stone/patient/year declined significantly in those treated with thiazides (mean difference (MD) −0.18, 95 % CI −0.30 to −0.06). Although follow-up was variable (from 5 months to 3 years), these findings support an important role for urinary Ca in Ca stone formation [21].

Finally, Strauss and colleagues further established a putative link between urinary Ca and Ca stone formation by demonstrating that medical therapy fails in patients with persistent hypercalciuria. Among 522 recurrent idiopathic Ca stone formers who entered a metabolic treatment program consisting of drug and dietary therapy, 57 patients demonstrated at least one recurrent stone and 189 remained free of new stones during a 2-year period. Mean urinary Ca was significantly higher in the group with recurrent stones compared to the group without recurrence (Ca 2.79±1.08 vs. 2.39±0.98 mg/kg/day, respectively), suggesting that idiopathic hypercalciuric stone formers with persistently high urinary Ca fail medical therapy [22].

## Restriction of Dietary Calcium

The impact of dietary Ca on urinary Ca and risk of stone formation has been the subject of intense debate. Historically, stone formers have been advised to reduce dietary Ca intake in an effort to reduce urinary Ca and decrease the risk of stone formation. However, recently investigators have questioned the effectiveness of dietary Ca restriction in reducing stone recurrence and have expressed additional concern about bone loss.

### *In Support of Calcium Restriction*

Dietary Ca impacts urinary Ca levels through two mechanisms. First, dietary Ca intake determines the filtered load of Ca: the more Ca ingested and absorbed, the higher the filtered load of Ca and the greater the urinary Ca excretion [23]. Second, the ingestion of Ca modulates serum Ca levels, altering the secretion of serum parathyroid hormone (PTH), which regulates renal tubular Ca reabsorption via a cyclic adenosine monophosphate (cAMP)-mediated pathway [24, 25].

Adams and colleagues demonstrated in 32 healthy volunteers that an increased Ca intake (administered as Ca carbonate) over a 4-day period was associated with a rise in serum Ca within 6 h, followed by an increase in urinary Ca, an immediate decline in serum PTH and urinary cAMP and an eventual fall in plasma vitamin D (1,25(OH)2D) within 18–24 h. Conversely, reduced Ca intake over 4 days resulted in an immediate decline in serum and urine Ca, an increase in PTH and urinary cAMP, and ultimately a rise in 1,25(OH)2D within 48 h [23]. In all, these findings suggest that short-term Ca restriction reduces urinary excretion of Ca by decreasing the filtered load of Ca and enhancing renal tubular reabsorption of Ca through upregulation of serum PTH and urinary cAMP. Based on these studies and others, restriction of dietary Ca was recommended for patients with kidney stones, particularly those with Ca stones and/or hypercalciuria, as a way to reduce urinary Ca and ostensibly stone risk. Notably, however, the long-term effects of increased or decreased Ca intake on intestinal Ca absorption and urinary Ca excretion were not explored in this study and the corresponding effects of Ca loading or deprivation on other urinary stone risk factors, such as oxalate, and urinary saturation of Ca stone-forming salts was not evaluated in this study.

## *Against Calcium Restriction*

Initial enthusiasm for dietary Ca restriction in stone formers was later tempered by an appreciation of the complexity of factors that contribute to urinary Ca and stone risk and because of concern that dietary Ca restriction may be detrimental to bone health. Dietary Ca, by way of downstream influences on PTH and vitamin D, exerts additional effects on organs outside the urinary tract, including bone, and the net effect of dietary Ca restriction on individuals with idiopathic hypercalciuria has not been completely elucidated.

Individuals with idiopathic hypercalciuria and stones demonstrate increased intestinal absorption of Ca and have been shown to excrete higher amounts of urinary Ca at any level of dietary Ca intake [26]. Furthermore, patients with idiopathic hypercalciuria maintained on restricted Ca diets were observed to excrete more Ca in the urine than they ingested, suggesting that bone resorption or alterations in renal tubular absorption of Ca may be at play [27]. Hence, simply decreasing dietary Ca intake may not substantially reduce urinary Ca excretion in some hypercalciuric stone formers.

Worcester and colleagues attempted to determine whether filtered load or renal tubular reabsorption of Ca plays the larger role in idiopathic hypercalciuria by comparing ten patients with idiopathic hypercalciuria to seven normocalciuric control subjects in a small metabolic study. Blood and urine samples were collected from the subjects while fasting and within 30–60 min of three meals over a 24 h period. In both cases and controls, urine Ca increased and fractional urinary reabsorption of Ca decreased with meals. However, the decline in urinary reabsorption of Ca was more pronounced in the hypercalciuric patients (adjusted mean=−0.024, 95 % CI −0.033 to −0.015) compared to the control subjects (adjusted mean=−0.010, 95 % CI −0.015 to −0.005). Interestingly, serum PTH did not significantly differ between the two groups [28]. These findings support reduced renal tubular Ca reabsorption as the primary means by which the kidneys excrete Ca into the urine postprandially, and while the exact mechanism was not determined, their data suggest that alterations in PTH alone fail to completely account for this response.

Dietary Ca restriction may increase the risk of stone formation through its interaction with other metabolic substrates that contribute to Ca stone formation, such as urinary oxalate, which will be reviewed in detail in the next section. Reduced dietary Ca intake may also be associated with an increase in protein consumption, which may potentiate the risk of stone formation by inducing hyperuricosuria, hypocitraturia, and low urinary pH [29].

A sustained low Ca diet can additionally lead to a negative Ca balance and the potential for bone demineralization. Idiopathic hypercalciuric patients have been shown to exhibit decreased bone mineral density, enhanced bone resorption, and reduced bone formation [30–32]. Additionally, hypercalciuric patients are at increased risk of bone fractures. Consequently, restricting dietary Ca may have a further deleterious effect on bone health. However, it has not been definitively established whether the increased fracture risk seen in hypercalciuric patients is related to the primary disorder that leads to stone formation or if it is a consequence of the negative Ca balance that occurs with decreased Ca intake in some patients in response to stone formation [31].

## *Calcium Oxalate Interaction*

The effect of dietary Ca on stone risk must take into account not only the effect on urinary Ca but also the effect on other urinary parameters that contribute to risk of stone formation. Ca and oxalate have an intricate relationship in the intestine that affects their respective intestinal absorption and urinary excretion, and ultimately stone formation (Fig. 3.1). The ratio of Ca to oxalate in the intestine has been shown to be an important factor in their solubility and absorption from the intestine, which in turn influences renal excretion.

Holmes and coworkers investigated the contribution of dietary oxalate to urinary oxalate excretion in 12 normal subjects without a history of stones who were provided controlled, solid food diets containing 10, 50, and 250 mg of oxalate/2,500 kcal. Overall, urinary oxalate increased as the oxalate content of the diets increased, with the mean contribution of dietary oxalate to urinary oxalate determined to be much higher than previous estimates, ranging from $24.4 \pm 15.5\%$ on the 10 mg/2,500 kcal/day diet to $41.5 \pm 9.1\%$ on the 250 mg/2,500 kcal/day diet. For subjects on the 250 mg oxalate diet, urinary oxalate excretion increased by a mean of $28.2 \pm 4.8\%$ and the dietary contribution to urinary oxalate increased to $52.6 \pm 8.6\%$ when the Ca content of the diet was reduced by 600 mg [33]. These findings suggest that up to half of urinary oxalate is derived from the diet, a much higher proportion than previously reported. The observed inverse relationship between dietary Ca and urinary oxalate is postulated to result from Ca-oxalate complex formation in the intestine, which reduces the amount of free oxalate available for absorption and ultimately urinary excretion (see Fig. 3.1).

Lange and colleagues further explored the interaction between Ca and oxalate by focusing on the ratio of Ca to oxalate at mealtime rather than on the daily consumption of each metabolite in order to determine effects on urinary excretion at distinct time points during the day rather than averaged over a 24-h collection. They studied ten healthy non-stone-forming adults in a two-phase metabolic study in which subjects consumed two different diets comprising 1,000 mg Ca and 750 mg oxalate in each 1-week phase. During one phase, the "balanced" meal plan, the content of Ca and oxalate were nearly equal at each of three daily meals, while in the second phase, an "imbalanced" meal plan provided 400 mg of Ca and 20 mg of oxalate for

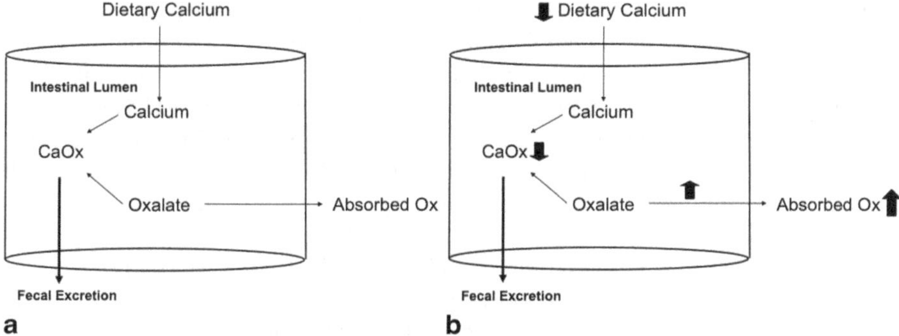


**Fig. 3.1** Calcium-oxalate interaction. **a**. In the setting of normal calcium intake, dietary calcium binds to oxalate in the intestinal lumen, forming a calcium-oxalate complex that is excreted in the stool. Unbound oxalate is absorbed from the intestine into the blood stream and ultimately excreted in the urine. **b** In the setting of low calcium intake, there is less calcium-oxalate complex formation, leaving a larger pool of luminal unbound oxalate to be absorbed into the bloodstream and excreted in the urine

breakfast and lunch and 200 mg of Ca and 710 mg of oxalate at dinner. Although total urinary Ca and oxalate, as well as Ca oxalate supersaturation, were comparable during the two meal plans, there were differences in urinary Ca and oxalate excretion at specific time intervals. Urinary Ca excretion was significantly lower on the balanced versus the imbalanced plan at the 1–6 pm (83.1 vs. 110.2 mg, respectively, $p < 0.04$) and 6–11 pm (71.3 vs. 107.2 mg, respectively, $p < 0.02$) time intervals, likely because the Ca content of the 8 am and 1 pm meals was higher on the imbalanced plan. Conversely, the 11 pm to 8 am urine collection on the imbalanced plan revealed lower urinary Ca than on the balanced plan (41.8 vs. 55.0 mg, respectively, $p < 0.02$), reflecting the lower Ca content of the evening meal on the imbalanced plan. Surprisingly, urinary oxalate was significantly higher on the balanced versus imbalanced diet at the 1–6 pm interval (28.1 vs. 16.7 mg, respectively, $p < 0.01$), despite ingestion of an oxalate load with the evening meal on the imbalanced plan. These findings reflect the complex interaction between Ca and oxalate as well as differences in the timing of their absorption, but they suggest that as long as the recommended daily amount of Ca is consumed, even relatively large amounts of oxalate may not significantly affect Ca oxalate stone risk [34].

## Dietary Calcium and Stone Risk

Support for avoidance of dietary Ca restriction in stone formers is derived from three large epidemiologic studies and a randomized trial. In a cohort of 45,619 male health-care professionals without a prior history of stones (HPFS), dietary Ca was assessed by way of semiquantitative food frequency questionnaires, which were administered at baseline and every 4 years thereafter, and subjects were queried about the occurrence of first-time, or incident, symptomatic kidney stones. Among 505 documented incident stones occurring during this period, 71 % of subjects with knowledge of their stone composition reported that their stones contained Ca. Mean daily dietary Ca intake was significantly lower in men who developed kidney stones compared to men without kidney stones ($797 \pm 280$ vs. $851 \pm 307$ mg, respectively, $p < 0.001$). On multivariate analyses a higher dietary Ca intake was associated with a reduced risk of kidney stones. After adjusting for potential confounding factors, men in the highest quintile of Ca intake had a 34 % lower rate of incident stones compared to those in the lowest quintile (95 % CI, 0.49–0.90, $p = 0.018$) [35].

Taylor and coworkers revisited this cohort of men after 14 years of follow-up and reexamined the relationship between dietary Ca intake and risk of incident, symptomatic kidney stones according to age [36]. For men under age 60, they found an inverse relationship between dietary Ca intake and risk of incident stones (multivariate RR 0.69, 95 % CI 0.56–0.87, $p = 0.01$ comparing those in the highest to those in the lowest quintile of Ca intake). In contrast, no association could be demonstrated between dietary Ca intake and risk of incident stones in men 60 years and older, suggesting that this association varies with age in men [36].

Curhan and colleagues found a similar relationship between dietary Ca intake and incident stone formation in two large female cohorts, older nurses (NHS I) and younger nurses (NHS II). New, symptomatic kidney stones were reported in 864 women in NHS I, with 86 % of stone forming subjects with a stone analysis reporting a Ca component to their stones. The multivariate relative risk of incident stones was 0.65 (95 % CI, 0.50–0.83, $p = 0.005$) in the highest quintile of Ca intake compared to the lowest [37]. Likewise, with 1,473 incident stone occurrences in NHS II, multivariate analyses revealed a relative risk reduction of 27 % (RR 0.73, 95 % CI, 0.59–0.90, $p = 0.007$) in the highest compared to the lowest quintile of Ca intake [38]. In all three large cohorts, the inverse relationship between dietary Ca intake and risk of incident kidney stone formation was attributed to the interaction between Ca and oxalate in the intestinal tract by which dietary Ca restriction reduces Ca oxalate complex formation, thereby increasing intestinal oxalate absorption and urinary excretion.

In an effort to characterize whether the source of dietary Ca intake (dairy or non-dairy) affects the relationship between dietary Ca intake and stone risk, Taylor and colleagues analyzed the association of dairy and non-dairy sources of Ca with symptomatic nephrolithiasis in the three large cohorts (excluding men 60 years and older in HPFS) [39]. On multivariable analysis, the relative risks of incident stone formation for subjects in the highest versus lowest quintiles of non-dairy Ca intake were 0.71 (95 % CI 0.56–0.92, $p = 0.007$) in HPFS, 0.82 (95 % CI 0.69–0.98, $p = 0.08$) in NHS I, and 0.74 (95 % CI 0.63–0.87, $p = 0.002$) in NHS II. Similar comparisons for dairy-based Ca intake revealed relative risks of 0.77 (95 % CI 0.63–0.95, $p = 0.01$) for HPFS, 0.83 (95 % CI 0.69–0.99, $p = 0.05$) for NHS I, and 0.76 (95 % CI 0.65–0.88, $p = 0.001$) for NHS II. These results suggest that the protective effect of dietary Ca against stone risk can be seen whether the Ca is derived from a dairy or non-dairy source [39].

A single RCT also examined the effect of dietary Ca on rate of recurrent kidney stones. Borghi and colleagues randomized 120 recurrent hypercalciuric Ca stone-forming men to a normal Ca, low animal protein, low sodium diet or a low Ca diet with no defined parameters for animal protein or sodium. After five years of follow-up they observed that the low Ca group had a significantly higher rate of stone recurrence than the normal Ca group (38 vs. 20%, respectively, RR=0.49, 95% CI 0.24–0.98, $p$=0.04). Urine Ca levels declined comparably between groups; however, urinary oxalate excretion increased in men on the low Ca diet by an average of 5.4 mg per day and decreased on the normal Ca diet by an average of 7.2 mg per day [40]. These findings support the results of the cohort studies and provide further evidence to discourage dietary Ca restriction in Ca stone formers. However, it is important to note that the independent effects of Ca, sodium, and animal protein on stone risk were not evaluated.

Fink and associates performed a systematic review and meta-analysis to evaluate the beneficial and adverse effects of drug, diet, and supplements on the secondary prevention of urinary stones. They identified three RCTs that examined the efficacy of multicomponent dietary intervention on stone recurrence rates but were unable to identify any trials that evaluated the independent effect of dietary Ca on risk of stone recurrence. However, based on the effect of individual dietary constituents from multicomponent diet intervention trials, the authors concluded that normal Ca intake lowered the risk of stone recurrence compared to a general or low Ca diet [41].

Although epidemiologic data and multicomponent dietary intervention trials provide compelling evidence to reverse the previous dogma that Ca stone formers, particularly hypercalciuric stone formers, should be advised to restrict dietary Ca, the issue is more complex. Curhan and coworkers obtained 24 h urine specimens from a subset of his large cohorts, including both those who did ($n$=807) and did not ($n$=239) form urinary stones during follow-up. Despite a decreasing risk of incident stones with increasing dietary Ca intake in these cohorts, the authors found that after adjusting for other confounding factors the relative risk of symptomatic incident stones increased with increasing urinary Ca (RR of stones in those with urinary Ca concentration $\geq$200 vs.$\leq$75 mg/L was 4.34, 95% CI 1.59–11.88 for older women; RR 51.09, 95% CI 4.27–611.1 for younger women; and RR 4.30, 95% CI 1.71–10.84 for men). Furthermore, mean 24 h urinary excretion of oxalate did not differ between those who did and did not form stones [19]. These findings validate the importance of urinary Ca in stone formation but fail to support the hypothesis that the increased risk of incident stone formation with low Ca intake is due to increased urinary oxalate excretion. Likewise, although Borghi and colleagues found that over time, the low Ca diet in their RCT was associated with a reduction in urinary Ca and an increase in urinary oxalate, they still noted an overall decrease in urinary saturation of Ca oxalate, which they attributed to a concomitant increase in urinary volume [40].

To further elucidate the relationship between Ca and oxalate intake and stone risk, Heller and colleagues performed a two-phase, randomized, crossover metabolic study in 21 normal subjects without a history of kidney stones in which they duplicated the diets of those in the highest and lowest quintiles of Ca intake described in Curhan's epidemiologic studies [35, 37, 42]. Because the oxalate content of these diets was not specified, the oxalate content of the controlled metabolic diet was set low at only 74–79 mg/day. Although urinary Ca, not surprisingly, was significantly higher compared to lower Ca diet (148 vs. 118 mg, respectively, $p < 0.01$), there was no significant difference in urinary oxalate or in urinary saturation of Ca oxalate between the two groups. These findings suggest that concomitant favorable changes in other urinary parameters associated with the high Ca diet, offset the increased propensity for Ca stone formation associated with an increase in urinary Ca. Indeed, evaluation of other urinary parameters revealed an increase in stone-protective factors, such as urine volume, potassium, phosphorous, pH, and citrate. After adjusting for other confounding factors, however, urinary saturation of Ca oxalate was higher on the high Ca diet than on the low Ca diet (5.6 vs. 4.5, respectively, $p = 0.03$) [42]. Consequently, although limiting dietary oxalate intake can avert the rise in urinary oxalate seen with dietary Ca restriction, other factors associated with a high Ca diet may provide a protective effect that can offset the increase in urinary Ca.

Curhan and colleagues also noted in their three large cohort studies that dietary Ca was not an independently changing parameter. Subjects in the higher quintiles of Ca intake also had higher levels of stone-protective factors, such as potassium, magnesium, phosphorus, and fluid [35, 37, 38]. Therefore, Ca, taken as food, may be associated with the coingestion of other stone-protective factors that contribute to the inverse relationship between dietary Ca and stone risk.

Matsumoto and coworkers further addressed the complex relationship between dietary and urinary Ca and oxalate in another two-phase metabolic study in ten normal, non-stone-forming subjects, similar to the study of Heller and coworkers [42]—except they imposed a liberal oxalate intake (200 mg/day) and varied only Ca between the two diets (1,000 mg/day in the normal Ca diet and 400 mg/day in the low Ca diet). They also detected a higher urinary Ca on the normal Ca versus low Ca diet (171 vs.124 mg/day, respectively, $p = 0.002$). However, urinary oxalate was higher during the low Ca phase compared to the normal Ca phase (27 vs. 25 mg/day, respectively, $p = 0.02$), likely due to enhanced intestinal absorption of oxalate during the low Ca diet, given adequate oxalate intake. However, urinary saturation of Ca oxalate was higher on the normal Ca diet than on the low Ca diet (4.3 vs. 3.5, respectively, $p = 0.0004$), even after adjusting for other urinary factors, suggesting that in the setting of liberal oxalate intake, although urinary Ca increases with a higher Ca intake, the decrease in urinary oxalate that is typically seen with a higher Ca intake does not overcome the effect of increased urinary Ca. Of note, the higher Ca diet in this study actually represents the recommended daily allowance (RDA) for Ca in men and younger woman, and therefore these data infer that in normal subjects, liberal oxalate consumption in the setting of the recommended Ca intake may enhance the risk of Ca oxalate stone formation [43].

Pak and colleagues investigated the effect of dietary Ca and oxalate restriction in a retrospective review of 951 stone formers from their metabolic clinic in whom 24 h urine studies were compared at baseline and after the initiation of moderate Ca and oxalate restriction during the initial comprehensive evaluation. Among patients with hypercalciuria at baseline, urinary Ca decreased by 29% in those with moderate–severe hypercalciuria, by 19% in those with mild hypercalciuria, and by 10% in normocalciuric patients. On the other hand, urinary oxalate did not change significantly from baseline in any of the three groups, and urinary saturation of Ca oxalate declined by 12, 6, and 0 %, respectively [44]. These findings also suggest that dietary oxalate restriction can prevent the rise in urinary oxalate associated with Ca restriction.

Finally, in a retrospective study of 28 recurrent hypercalciuric stone formers, Pak and coworkers showed that the combined effect of dietary modifications (modest Ca and oxalate restriction) and pharmacotherapy (thiazide diuretics/indapamide and potassium citrate) resulted in a significant decrease in urinary Ca from baseline (346 –248 mg/day, respectively, $p=0.001$) without a rise in urinary oxalate. Additionally, stone formation rate nearly ceased and bone mineral density at the lumbar spine and the femoral neck significantly improved over the mean 3.7 years of follow-up [45].

In summary, these studies suggest that although a higher Ca intake in the setting of either low or high oxalate intake can increase urinary Ca, the concomitant intake of stone-protective factors such as fluid and alkali as well as the reduction in urinary oxalate may at least partially offset the risk conferred by increased urinary Ca, although this has never been studied in a prospective, long-term trial. On the other hand, dietary Ca restriction must be accompanied by oxalate restriction in order to potentially reduce stone risk. Mild dietary Ca and oxalate restriction, along with pharmacologic hypocalciuric agents, can reduce stone risk without comprising bone mineral density. Unfortunately, the Borghi trial [40] did not specifically compare normal and low Ca diets in the setting of oxalate restriction in the absence of other variables; therefore, it is not clear if mild Ca restriction along with oxalate restriction is as effective as normal Ca, low sodium, low animal protein intake in reducing stone risk and maintaining bone mineral density without additional pharmacologic agents. Consequently, at this time, normal Ca intake (the RDA), along with mild oxalate restriction, is recommended to prevent stones and preserve bone health.

## Calcium Supplementation

Ca supplementation is increasingly recommended, particularly for older woman, to improve bone health. However, the form in which Ca is administered, either as food or supplement, has been shown to differentially influence stone risk. Ca supplementation was one of the factors evaluated for effect on incident, symptomatic kidney stone formation in the large cohort studies. In older woman (NHS I, women age 30–55), but not in men (HPFS) or younger women (NHS II), multivariate analysis revealed an increased risk of stone formation associated with use of 1–100 mg of supplemental Ca daily compared to no supplemental Ca (RR 1.26 (CI, 0.79–2.00)), with no additional risk appreciated in women who consumed more than this amount daily [35, 38].

In the largest study to date analyzing the risk of stone formation with use of supplemental Ca, the Women's Health Initiative (WHI) randomized 36,282 postmenopausal women to 1,000 mg of Ca carbonate and 400 IU vitamin $D_3$ daily or to placebo, with a primary endpoint of the rate of hip fractures. However, subjects were additionally queried annually about new stone events as part of the adverse events reporting. A total of 449 women in the intervention group versus 381 women in the placebo group reported having a stone, translating into a 17 % higher risk of kidney stones in the Ca and vitamin D group compared to the control group [46]. Wallace et al. revisited the WHI data in an attempt to identify a reason for the increased risk of stones seen in the Ca and vitamin D group, but were unable to identify either baseline patient characteristics or dietary habits that could account for the increased risk of kidney stones other than use of Ca and vitamin D supplementation [47]. Of note, however, women taking Ca supplements at baseline were not required to discontinue the supplements while enrolled in the study. In both groups, 65 % of participants reported a baseline daily Ca intake of approximately 800 mg, and consequently, those randomly assigned to receive an additional 1,000 mg of Ca daily raised their total Ca intake to upwards of 1,800 mg/day, despite an RDA for Ca of 1,100 to 1,200 mg daily.

Curhan and colleagues attributed the apparent contradiction between the effect of dietary Ca and supplemental Ca on stone risk by the timing of Ca supplementation [37]. Among women taking supplements in NHS I, 81 % took their Ca supplement apart from meals or at breakfast, a meal typically low in oxalate. By taking supplemental Ca outside of mealtime or with a low oxalate meal, the benefit of Ca in binding intestinal oxalate and reducing oxalate absorption is potentially lost.

Domrongkitchaiporn and colleagues explored the effect of timing of Ca supplementation on urinary stone risk in a two-phase metabolic crossover study in 32 men without a history of stones in whom 3 g of Ca carbonate was administered daily, either all at once at bedtime or as 1 g with each meal. Although urinary Ca excretion increased significantly from baseline in both groups, urinary oxalate declined only in the group taking Ca with meals (from 0.17 to 0.13 mmol/day, $p=0.01$) and not in those taking it at bedtime (from 0.15 to 0.15 mmol/day, $p=0.9$). Consequently, the activity product of Ca oxalate (an estimate of stone-forming risk) increased significantly when Ca was taken at bedtime (from 0.47 to 0.72, $p<0.01$) but not when it was taken with meals (0.54–0.57, $p=0.54$) [48]. Thus, the increase in urinary Ca seen with Ca supplementation is offset by a reduction in urinary oxalate only when the supplements are taken at mealtime.

In summary, if Ca supplementation is necessary (in those unable to ingest the recommended daily allowance of dietary Ca), the supplements should be taken with a meal that is likely to contain higher amounts of oxalate, such as lunch or dinner.

## Conclusion

Recommendations for stone formers regarding dietary Ca intake must take into account not only the effect of Ca on stone formation but also the effect on bone mineral density. There is consensus among stakeholders that severe Ca restriction should be avoided. Furthermore, it is clear that dietary oxalate intake modulates the effect of dietary Ca on stone risk, and modest oxalate intake is advisable. Although higher dietary Ca intake increases urinary Ca and presumably increases stone risk, the combined effect of potentially lowering urinary oxalate and favorably changing other stone risk factors with the coingestion of stone-protective foods may offset the effect of increasing urinary Ca and overall lower stone risk. Dietary Ca recommendations should follow the recommended daily allowance, but should not exceed it, and taking Ca as food rather than supplement should be encouraged. For stone formers with reduced bone mineral density, who are unable to achieve the RDA of Ca intake due to intolerance of dairy or non-dairy Ca sources, judicious Ca supplementation at lunch or dinner can be cautiously undertaken. Finally, close monitoring of 24-h urine parameters during treatment should help guide dietary and pharmacological recommendations so that adjustments can be made preemptively before actual stone recurrence is realized.

# References


1. Stamatelou KK, Francis ME, Jones CA, Nyberg LM, Curhan GC. Time trends in reported prevalence of kidney stones in the United States: 1976–1994. Kidney Int. 2003 May;63(5):1817–23.
2. Peterson AC, Curtis LH, Shea AM, Borawski KM, Schulman KA, Scales CD Jr. Urinary diversion in patients with spinal cord injury in the United States. Urology. 2012 Dec;80(6):1247–51.
3. Ljunghall S, Danielson BG. A prospective study of renal stone recurrences. Br J Urol. 1984 April;56(2):122–4.
4. Trinchieri A, Ostini F, Nespoli R, Rovera F, Montanari E, Zanetti G. A prospective study of recurrence rate and risk factors for recurrence after a first renal stone. J Urol. 1999 July;162(1):27–30.
5. Pearle MS, Calhoun EA, Curhan GC, Urologic Diseases of America Project, et al. Urologic diseases in America project: urolithiasis. J Urol. 2005 March;173(3):848–57.
6. Saigal CS, Joyce G, Timilsina AR. Urologic Diseases in America Project: direct and indirect costs of nephrolithiasis in an employed population: opportunity for disease management? Kidney Int. 2005 Oct;68(4):1808–14.
7. Pak CY. Should patients with single renal stone occurrence undergo diagnostic evaluation? J Urol. 1982 May;127(5):855–58.
8. Coe FL, Parks JH, Asplin JR. The pathogenesis and treatment of kidney stones. N Engl J Med. 1992 Oct 15;327(16):1141–52.
9. Bushinsky DA. Nephrolithiasis. J Am Soc Nephrol. 1998 May;9(5):917–24.
10. Wilson DM. Clinical and laboratory approaches for evaluation of nephrolithiasis. J Urol. 1989 March;141(3 Pt 2):770.
11. Pak CY, Britton F, Peterson R, Ward D, Northcutt C, Breslau NA, et al. Ambulatory evaluation of nephrolithiasis: classification, clinical presentation and diagnostic criteria. Am J Med. 1980 July;69(1):19–30.
12. Hodgkinson A, Pyrah LN. The urinary excretion of calcium and inorganic phosphate in 344 patients with calcium stone of renal origin. Br J Surg. 1958 July;46(195):10–8.
13. Parks JH, Coe FL. A urinary calcium-citrate index for the evaluation of nephrolithiasis. Kidney Int. 1986 July;30(1):85.
14. Menon M. Calcium oxalate renal lithiasis: endocrinology and metabolism. In: Rajfer J, editor. Urologic endocrinology. Philadelphia: Saunders; 1986 p. 386.

15. Pak CY, Oata M, Lawrence EC, Snyder W. The hypercalciurias. Causes, parathyroid functions, and diagnostic criteria. J Clin Invest. 1974 Aug;54(2):387–400.
16. Worcester EM, Coe FL. Clinical practice. Calcium kidney stones. N Engl J Med. 2010 Sep 2;363(10):954–63.
17. Albright F, Henneman P, Benedict PH, Forbes AP. Idiopathic hypercalciuria: a preliminary report. Proc R Soc Med. 1953 Dec;46(12):1077–81.
18. Worcester EM, Coe FL. New insights into the pathogenesis of idiopathic hypercalciuria. Semin Nephrol. 2008 Mar;28(2):120–32.
19. Curhan GC, Willett WC, Speizer FE, Stampfer MJ. Twenty-four-hour urine chemistries and the risk of kidney stones among women and men. Kidney Int. 2001 June;59(6):2290–8.
20. Pearle MS, Roehrborn CG, Pak CY. Meta-analysis of randomized trials for medical prevention of calcium oxalate nephrolithiasis. J Endourol. 1999 Nov;13(9):679–85.
21. Escribano J, Balaguer A, Pagone F, Feliu A, Roqué I Figuls M. Pharmacological interventions for preventing complications in idiopathic hypercalciuria. Cochrane Database Syst Rev. 2009;(1):CD004754.
22. Strauss AL, Coe FL, Deutsch L, Parks JH. Factors that predict relapse of calcium nephrolithiasis during treatment: a prospective study. Am J Med. 1982 Jan;72(1):17–24.
23. Adams ND, Gray RW, Lemann J Jr. The effects of oral CaCO3 loading and dietary calcium deprivation on plasma 1,25-dihydroxyvitamin D concentrations in healthy adults. J Clin Endocrinol Metab. 1979 June;48(6):1008–16.
24. Widrow SH, Levinsky NG. The effect of parathyroid extract on renal tubular calcium reabsorption in the dog. J Clin Invest. 1962 Dec;41:2151–9.
25. Agus ZS, Gardner LB, Beck LH, Goldberg M. Effects of parathyroid hormone on renal tubular reabsorption of calcium, sodium, and phosphate. Am J Physiol. 1973 May;224(5):1143–8.
26. Bleich HL, Moore MJ, Lemann J Jr, Adams ND, Gray RW. Urinary calcium excretion in human beings. N Engl J Med. 1979 Sep 6;301(10):535–41
27. Coe FL, Favus MJ, Crockett T, Strauss AL, Parks JH, Porat A, et al. Effects of low-calcium diet on urine calcium excretion, parathyroid function and serum 1,25(OH)2D3 levels in patients with idiopathic hypercalciuria and in normal subjects. Am J Med. 1982 Jan;72(1):25–32.
28. Worcester EM, Gillen DL, Evan AP, Parks JH, Wright K, Trumbore L et al. Evidence that postprandial reduction of renal calcium reabsorption mediates hypercalciuria of patients with calcium nephrolithiasis. Am J Physiol Renal Physiol. 2007 Jan;292(1):66–75.
29. Borghi L, Meschi T, Maggiore U, Prati B. Dietary therapy in idiopathic nephrolithiasis. Nutr Rev. 2006 July;64(7 Pt 1):301–12.
30. Gomes SA, dos Reis LM, Noronha IL, Jorgetti V, Heilberg IP. RANKL is a mediator of bone resorption in idiopathic hypercalciuria. Clin J Am Soc Nephrol. 2008 Sep;3(5):1446–52.
31. Heilberg IP, Weisinger JR. Bone disease in idiopathic hypercalciuria. Curr Opin Nephrol Hypertens. 2006 July;15(4):394–402.
32. Heller HJ, Zerwekh JE, Gottschalk FA, Pak CY. Reduced bone formation and relatively increased bone resorption in absorptive hypercalciuria. Kidney Int. 2007 April;71(8):808–15.
33. Holmes RP, Goodman HO, Assimos DG. Contribution of dietary oxalate to urinary oxalate excretion. Kidney Int. 2001 Jan;59(1):270–6.
34. Lange JN, Wood KD, Mufarrij PW, Callahan MF, Easter L, Knight J, et al. The impact of dietary calcium and oxalate ratios on stone risk. Urology. 2012 June;79(6):1226–9.
35. Curhan GC, Willett WC, Rimm EB, Stampfer MJ. A prospective study of dietary calcium and other nutrients and the risk of symptomatic kidney stones. N Engl J Med. 1993 March 25;328(12):833–8.
36. Taylor EN, Stampfer MJ, Curhan GC. Dietary factors and the risk of incident kidney stones in men: new insights after 14 years of follow-up. J Am Soc Nephrol. 2004 Dec;15(12):3225–32.
37. Curhan GC, Willett WC, Speizer FE, Spiegelman D, Stampfer MJ. Comparison of dietary calcium with supplemental calcium and other nutrients as factors affecting the risk for kidney stones in women. Ann Intern Med. 1997 April 1;126(7):497–504.

38. Curhan GC, Willett WC, Knight EL, Stampfer MJ. Dietary factors and the risk of incident kidney stones in younger women: Nurses' Health Study II. Arch Intern Med. 2004 April 26;164(8):885–95.
39. Taylor EN, Curhan GC. Dietary calcium from dairy and nondairy sources, and risk of symptomatic kidney stones. J Urol. 2013 October;190(4):1255–9.
40. Borghi L, Schianchi T, Meschi T, Guerra A, Allegri F, Maggiore U, et al. Comparison of two diets for the prevention of recurrent stones in idiopathic hypercalciuria. N Engl J Med. 2002 Jan 10;346(2):77–84.
41. Fink HA, Akornor JW, Garimella PS, MacDonald R, Cutting A, Rutks IR et al. Diet, fluid, or supplements for secondary prevention of nephrolithiasis: a systematic review and meta-analysis of randomized trials. Eur Urol. 2009 July;56(1):72–80.
42. Heller HJ, Doerner MF, Brinkley LJ, Adams-Huet B, Pak CY. Effect of dietary calcium on stone forming propensity. J Urol. 2003 Feb;169(2):470–4.
43. Matsumoto ED, Heller IIJ, Adams-Huet B, Brinkley LJ, Pak CY, Pearle MS. Effect of high and low calcium diets on stone forming risk during liberal oxalate intake. J Urol. 2006 July;176(1):132–6.
44. Pak CY, Odvina CV, Pearle MS, Sakhaee K, Peterson RD, Poindexter JR, et al. Effect of dietary modification on urinary stone risk factors. Kidney Int. 2005 Nov;68(5):2264–73.
45. Pak CY, Heller HJ, Pearle MS, Odvina CV, Poindexter JR, Peterson RD, et al. Prevention of stone formation and bone loss in absorptive hypercalciuria by combined dietary and pharmacological interventions. J Urol. 2003 Feb;169(2):465–9.
46. Jackson RD, LaCroix AZ, Gass M, Wallace RB, Robbins J, Lewis CE, et al. Calcium plus vitamin D supplementation and the risk of fractures. N Engl J Med. 2006 Feb 16;354(7):669–83.
47. Wallace RB, Wactawski-Wende J, O'Sullivan MJ, Larson JC, Cochrane B, Gass M, et al. Urinary tract stone occurrence in the Women's Health Initiative (WHI) randomized clinical trial of calcium and vitamin D supplements. Am J Clin Nutr. 2011 Jul;94(1):270–7.
48. Domrongkitchaiporn S, Sopassathit W, Stitchantrakul W, Prapaipanich S, Ingsathit A, Rajatanavin R. Schedule of taking calcium supplement and the risk of nephrolithiasis. Kidney Int. 2004 May;65(5):1835–41.

# Chapter 4
# Citrus Juices and Prevention of Calcium Stones: Some, but Not All?

Michael P. Kurtz and Brian H. Eisner

## Background and Physiology

Citrate is a naturally occurring inhibitor of urinary stone formation. The mechanisms of citrate metabolism were discovered and reported by Hans Adolf Krebs in 1937 for which he was awarded the 1953 Nobel Prize in Physiology or Medicine. Low urine citrate (i.e., hypocitraturia) is a common finding among patients with calcium nephrolithiasis and may be present in 20–60 % of stone formers [1, 2]. Citrate inhibits stone formation through several pathways: It complexes with calcium, decreasing tubular concentration of calcium; it inhibits nucleation of calcium oxalate and calcium phosphate stones; it prevents crystal agglomeration in vitro; and it may prevent adhesion of calcium oxalate to renal epithelial cells [3]. As an organic anion, it represents potential base, as its hepatic and renal metabolism consumes a proton. Its administration is therefore associated with an increase in urine pH and inhibition of urate and cystine crystallization. Hypocitraturia is defined as <320 mg/day of citrate excreted in the urine [3].

Citrate excretion is determined mainly by the acid–base state of the patient in addition to oral intake of citrate. Acidosis decreases citrate synthesis in the peritubular cells and also enhances tubular resorption of citrate [4]. Hypocitraturia may develop through several means. Distal renal tubular acidosis (RTA) may cause a hyperchloremic acidosis associated with hypokalemia. Very low urinary citrate levels often accompany acidosis. Any condition that causes systemic acidosis may reduce citrate, such as chronic diarrheal states causing intestinal alkali wasting, high-protein or high-sodium diet, strenuous exercise, drugs that cause either extracellular fluid volume depletion or inhibit carbonic anhydrase, or advanced chronic kidney disease with impaired ability to excrete an acid load [4]. Genetic factors play a role, as vitamin D receptor and sodium dicarboxylate cotransporter polymorphisms are found at higher frequency in hypocitraturic stone formers than in normocitraturic stone formers and control populations [5]. Whether racial or ethnic differences may play

B. H. Eisner (✉) · M. P. Kurtz
Department of Urology, Massachusetts General Hospital, GRB 1102, 55 Fruit Street, Boston, MA 02114, USA
e-mail: beisner@partners.org

M. S. Pearle, S. Y. Nakada (eds.), *Practical Controversies in Medical Management of Stone Disease,* DOI 10.1007/978-1-4614-9575-8_4,

© Springer Science+Business Media New York 2014

a role is an emerging area of research, as there may be differences between Asian and white stone formers [6].

Pharmacological therapy is the current gold standard for hypocitraturic calcium nephrolithiasis. Pharmacological supplementation of citrate (with potassium citrate or potassium magnesium citrate) has been shown to significantly decrease stone recurrence when compared to placebo, both for patients with hypocitraturic calcium oxalate nephrolithiasis and in unselected calcium oxalate stone formers. Long-term efficacy was shown by Pak et al. in 1985; 89 patients with hypocitraturic calcium nephrolithiasis were given 60 mEq of potassium citrate daily (divided into three doses), and a nearly 80 % decrease in the need for surgical intervention was reported [7]. Alkali citrate supplementation has also been shown to be effective at promoting stone clearance and preventing recurrence in adults [8] and children [9] who have undergone shock wave lithotripsy (SWL).

Gastrointestinal side effects are not uncommon, though they may be mollified by taking citrate with meals [10]. There are potential metabolic side effects of medical therapy; the cation administered with citrate is either potassium or sodium. Potassium may result in hyperkalemia if administered to people with reduced glomerular filtration rate or those taking angiotensin-converting enzyme inhibitors or angiotensin receptor blockers. Sodium citrate is less likely than sodium chloride to cause worsening hypertension or edema in stone formers and is generally well tolerated. A prescription of Urocit-K 20 mEq involves taking two 1,080-mg tablets three times per day and costs between roughly US\$ 160–210 per month [11, 12]. As few as one in four patients may be closely adherent to the prescribed regimen [13]. When surveyed, patients appear to prefer dietary therapy to pharmacologic intervention [14, 15]. Tiselius polled 100 consecutive patients undergoing intervention for stones in Sweden. He found that 95 patients were motivated to change their dietary habits, whereas only 71 desired pharmacologic therapy. Similar results were found in 198 patients surveyed in a stone treatment center in Colorado in which 96 % of first-time stone formers and 97 % of recurrent stone formers were willing to modify their diet. By comparison, 86 and 87 % of first-time and recurrent stone formers were willing to take medications, though it is not stated if these differences were statistically different [15].

In 1996, Seltzer et al. published the first manuscript on manipulation of 24-h urine composition using a beverage; half a cup of concentrated lemon juice was mixed with seven and a half cups of water to make a "sugar-free lemonade." Urine citrate increased by a mean of 204 mg/day in 12 patients with hypocitraturic calcium oxalate nephrolithiasis [3].

## Water

Whereas the focus of this chapter is on fruit juices and other beverages that may alter urine citrate and kidney stone risk, it is important to acknowledge the effects of urinary volume and water intake on stone risk and recurrence. Borghi et al. performed a 5-year-randomized prospective study that enrolled 300 patients (calcium oxalate stone formers and controls) and demonstrated that fluid intake comprising volumes of >2 L significantly reduced stone risk and recurrence when compared with fluid volumes of 1 L [16]. These experimental findings have been corroborated in prospective epidemiologic cohort studies that have shown that increased fluid intake in men and women is associated with decreased risk of nephrolithiasis [17, 18].

## Citrate Content of Fruit Juices and Beverages

The 1986 food tables report the citric acid content (mg of citric acid per kg) of fruit in descending order: lemon, 49.2; grapefruit, 13.7; cranberry, 11; and orange, 10.6 [39]. A more recent nuclear magnetic resonance (NMR)-based study showed the following citrate levels (mmol/L) in descending order: grapefruit, 64.7; lemon, 47.6; orange, 38.7; cranberry, 19 [39]. These authors also reported the citrate content of various other beverages (grapefruit juice (Ruby Red), orange juice, pineapple juice, cranberry juice (Crystal Light), and lemon-flavored Gatorade, all have been shown to have greater amounts of citrate than lemonade). Using an enzyme-spectrophotometric method, Yilmaz et al. found similar results for stored lemon (37.5 mmol/L) and orange juices (36.0 mmol/L), but found that tomato juice had the highest citrate concentration (77.7 mmol/L) [40]. Tomato juice has greater amounts of citrate than lemon juice or orange juice, and this composition is conserved across at least three different species of tomato [41]. It is also a source of potassium at approximately 31 mEq/L, and low in sodium (100 mg/L) if no additional salt is added. These data have laid much of the groundwork for hypotheses and studies regarding the use of juices and beverages to supplement citrate and reduce kidney stone risk. However, it is important to note that total citrate was reported in the aforementioned publications, not citrate as alkali, which as described in the introduction is the key factor in determining whether the ingestion of a given beverage will result in citraturia. A single study examined the levels of citrate bound to alkali in diet sodas and demonstrated that some diet sodas will contain similar amounts of citrate as alkali to the original lemonade formula reported by Seltzer et al. [3, 38]. Tables 4.1, 4.2, and 4.3 list studies published in the English literature, caloric content, and citrate content of beverages, all of which are summarized in this chapter. Of note, citrate content is reported as total citrate, not citrate-as-alkali, as many of these studies did not report/calculate the total alkali content of the beverages that were studied.

## Lemonade

The most commonly studied beverage therapy for nephrolithiasis is lemonade. This has been studied in both hypocitraturic calcium stone formers and unselected calcium stone formers. Seltzer et al. in 1996 first reported that a "homemade lemonade" consisting of ~120 mL of reconstituted lemon juice (ReaLemon, Dr. Pepper Snapple

**Table 4.1** Studies in patients with a history of calcium stones

| Study | Formulation | N | Methodology | Total citrate intake daily | Caloric intake (estimated kcal) | Outcome (Δ urinary citrate), 24-h urine unless otherwise specified |
|---|---|---|---|---|---|---|
| *Lemon juice/lemonade* | | | | | | |
| Aras 2008 [19] | 85 mL fresh lemon juice and 1 L tap water per day | 20 | Patients with hypocitraturic nephrolithiasis; comparing intervention versus own baseline | 60 mEq | 21 kcal | 146 % increase; $p<0.003$ |
| Odvina 2006 [20] | 1.2 L reconstituted frozen lemonade in distilled water divided TID | 14 | Mixed cohort of healthy volunteers and calcium stone formers; crossover design | 100 mEq | 480 kcal | No change; $p>0.05$ |
| Penniston 2007 [21] | 118 mL lemon juice diluted with 828 mL water or 946 mL lemonade | 63 | Patients with calcium oxalate nephrolithiasis. Lemonade from concentrate or low-calorie commercially available lemonade | ~80 mEq | Unknown (>30 kcal) | No sustained change; $p>0.15$ |
| *Lime juice/limeade* | | | | | | |
| da Cunha 2012 [22] | 75 mL freshly squeezed lime juice and sucralose diluted in 310 mL water, single dose | 10 | Hypocirtaturic calcium-stone-forming patients. Citrate measured 2 h after a single juice bolus | 8.1 mEq | 173 kcal | 160 % increase; measured 2 h after juice ingestion in 2-h collection |
| *Orange juice* | | | | | | |
| da Cunha 2012 [22] | 385 mL freshly squeezed orange juice, single dose | 10 | Hypocirtaturic calcium-stone-forming patients. Citrate measured 2 h after a single juice bolus | 17.3 mEq | 19 kcal | 129 % increase; measured 2 h after juice ingestion in 2-h collection |
| *Cranberry juice* | | | | | | |
| Gettman 2005 [23] | 1 L Ocean Spray cranberry juice | 24 | 12 CaOx stone formers and 12 controls, pre/post intervention, 1 L cranberry juice vs. 1 L deionized water | 33.4 mEq | 535 kcal | No effect on citrate ($p=0.5$); increased urine oxalate and calcium |

**Table 4.1** (continued)

| Study | Formulation | N | Methodology | Total citrate intake daily | Caloric intake (estimated kcal) | Outcome ($\Delta$ urinary citrate), 24-h urine unless otherwise specified |
|---|---|---|---|---|---|---|
| *Carbonated and sports drinks* | | | | | | |
| Karagülle 2007 [24] | 1.5 L of carbonated water divided in four portions | 34 | Patients with known recurrent calcium oxalate stones and urine pH<6.3; comparison between groups given carbonated water either high or low in bicarbonate (99 mg/L vs. 2.67 mg/L) | None | 0 kcal | Decrease in citrate (9%) in higher bicarbonate group, but greater decrease in controls (33%); $p=0.03$ |
| *Miscellaneous* | | | | | | |
| da Cunha 2012 [22] | 300 mL freshly blended cantaloupe juice diluted in 85 mL of water, single dose | 10 | Hypocirtaturic calcium-stone-forming patients. Citrate measured 4 h after a single juice bolus | 17.3 mEq | 19 kcal | 59% increase; measured 4 h after juice ingestion in 2-h collection |

**Table 4.2** Studies in patients with a history of stones, type unspecified

| Study | Formulation | $n$ | Methodology | Total citrate intake daily | Caloric intake (estimated kcal) | Outcome ($\Delta$ urinary citrate), 24-h urine unless otherwise specified |
|---|---|---|---|---|---|---|
| *Lemon juice/lemonade* | | | | | | |
| Koff et al. [25] | 90 mL concentrated ReaLemon® and 531 mL water plus sweetener, divided into three portions daily | 21 | Patients with a history of nephrolithiasis; crossover design with 60 mEq K-Citrate | 63 mEq | 23 kcal+sweetener | No change; $p$ value not calculated |
| Kang 2007 [26] | 120 mL of concentrated lemon juice mixed with 2,000 mL tap water | 11 | Patient with hypocitraturic nephrolithiasis, eight glasses of lemonade solution/day (three glasses in the morning, two afternoon, three evening); pre vs. post analysis | 84 mEq | 30 kcal | 109 % increase; $p<0.05$ |
| *Lime juice/limeade* | | | | | | |
| Tosukhowong 2008 [27] | Hand-squeezed limes, freeze-dried, potassium added, diluted in 200 mL of tap water | 20 | 13 patients with history of urolithiasis assigned lime formulation; seven control patients taking lactose in 200 mL tap water | 63 mEq | 50 kcal | 383 % increase; $p=0.002$ |
| *Orange juice* | | | | | | |
| Wabner 1993 [28] | 1.2 L reconstituted frozen orange juice in distilled water divided TID | 11 | 11 individuals with hypocitraturic nephrolithiasis. Placebo phase, 1.2 L orange juice phase, and potassium citrate tablet phase | 190 mEq | 550 kcal | 67 % increase; $p<0.002$ |
| *Miscellaneous* | | | | | | |
| Taylor 2013 [29] | Nondairy animal protein (per 10 g/day) | 2,561 | Cross-sectional study of diet in three large prospective cohorts; 60 % of patients were stone formers | n/a | 40 kcal/10 g serving | 0.104 mEq/day decrease (0.057–0.15 95 % CI) per 10 g protein |
| – | Potassium (per 1,000 mg/day) | 2,561 | Cross-sectional study of diet in three large prospective cohorts; 60 % of patients were stone formers | n/a | n/a | 0.276 mEq/day increase (0.17–0.39 95 % CI) per 1,000 mg potassium |

**Table 4.2** (continued)

| Study | Formulation | n | Methodology | Total citrate intake daily | Caloric intake (estimated kcal) | Outcome (Δ urinary citrate), 24-h urine unless otherwise specified |
|---|---|---|---|---|---|---|
| – | Vitamin C (per 250/mg/day) | 2,561 | Cross-sectional study of diet in three large prospective cohorts; 60% of patients were stone formers | n/a | n/a | 0.026 mEq/day decrease (−0.005–0.062 95% CI) per 250 mg Vitamin C |
| Taylor 2009 [30] | Dietary approaches to stop hypertension (DASH diet) | 1,046 | Examination of diet in three large prospective cohorts; 60% of patients were stone formers | n/a | n/a | C12.2–16.9% increase between the lowest and highest quintiles, cohort dependent |

**Table 4.3** Studies in healthy volunteers or nonstone formers

| Study | Formulation | $n$ | Methodology | Total citrate intake daily | Caloric intake (estimated kcal) | Outcome ($\Delta$ urinary citrate), 24-h urine unless otherwise specified |
|---|---|---|---|---|---|---|
| *Lemon juice/lemonade* | | | | | | |
| Khan 2010 [31] | 60 mL concentrated lemon juice diluted 1,000 mL | 24 | Patients with an indwelling bladder catheter and history of catheter blockage | ~40 mEq | 22 kcal | 51 % increase; $p=0.001$ |
| *Orange juice* | | | | | | |
| Honow 2003 [32] | 500 mL or 1,000 mL orange juice from Krings, Herrath vs. mineral water | 9 | Healthy female volunteers, compared with controls | 23.3 (500 mL daily intake) or 46.7 (1,000 mL daily intake) | 224 kcal (500 mL daily intake) or 448 kcal (1,000 mL daily intake) estimated | 21.1 % increase (500 mL daily intake) $p<0.05$; 35.7 % increase (1,000 mL daily intake); $p<0.05$ |
| *Cranberry juice* | | | | | | |
| Kessler 2002 [33] | 330 mL cranberry juice diluted with up to 420 mL water | 12 | Healthy volunteers, up to 750 mL diluted cranberry juice. Comparison vs. mineral water | 17.2 mEq | 116 kcal | 10.6 % decrease; $p=$NS |
| McHarg 2003 [34] | Intake of 2 L tap water versus 500 mL cranberry/blended juice diluted 1:3 in tap water | 20 | 500 mL blended cranberry juice+1,500 mL tap water | Unable TBD (juice derived from mixture of grape/cranberry juices) | 359 kcal | 31 % increase in urinary citrate ($p<0.001$) |
| *Grapefruit juice* | | | | | | |
| Honow 2003 [32] | 500 mL or 1,000 mL Grapefruit juice from "master product" (Hamburger Warencenter, Hamburgh, Germany) vs. mineral water | 9 | Healthy female volunteers, compared with controls | 36.7 (500 mL daily intake) or 73.4 (1,000 mL daily intake) | 196.5 kcal (500 mL daily intake) or 393 kcal (1,000 mL daily intake) estimated | 20.5 % increase (500 mL daily intake) $p<0.05$; 47.6 % increase (1,000 mL daily intake); $p<0.01$ |

**Table 4.3** (continued)

| Study | Formulation | n | Methodology | Total citrate intake daily | Caloric intake (estimated kcal) | Outcome ($\Delta$ urinary citrate), 24-h urine unless otherwise specified |
|---|---|---|---|---|---|---|
| Goldfarb 2001 [35] | 720 mL Tropicana brand grapefruit juice | 10 | Ten healthy volunteers, 720 mL tap water vs. 720 mL grapefruit juice | 46 mEq | 270 kcal | 17 % increase; $p<0.05$ |
| *Carbonated and sports drinks* | | | | | | |
| Goodman et al. 2009 [36] | 946 mL Performance (Shacklee Corporation) | 16 | Healthy volunteers; six in Gatorade arm, six in Performance arm, four in both. one quart per day of each. Tap water control | 18 mEq | 400 kcal | Increase 30 % ($p=0.003$) |
| – | 946 mL Gatorade Thirst Quencher Original (Gatorade) | 16 | Healthy volunteers; six in Gatorade arm, six in Performance arm, four in both. one quart per day of each. Tap water control | 13 mEq | 200 kcal | No significant change (7.9 % increase, but $p>0.05$) |
| Passman et al. 2009 [37] | Diet Coke | 6 | Six healthy volunteers drank water, caffeine-free Diet Coke®, and Fresca® separated by washout periods | 0.78 mEq/L | 0 | No significant change (16.7 % (increase, but $p>0.05$) |
| – | Fresca | 6 | Six healthy volunteers drank water, caffeine-free Diet Coke, and Fresca separated by washout periods | 12.1 mEq/L | 0 | No significant change (6.37 % increase, but $p>0.05$) |

**Table 4.3** (continued)

| Study | Formulation | n | Methodology | Total citrate intake daily | Caloric intake (estimated kcal) | Outcome (Δ urinary citrate), 24-h urine unless otherwise specified |
|---|---|---|---|---|---|---|
| Sumorok et al. 2012 [38] | Diet Sunkist Orange Soda | 9 | Healthy volunteers. Water intake compared with three cans of Diet Sunkist Orange soda per day | 8.88 mEq/day of citrate as alkali | 0 | No difference detected; 95% CI ($-75$–195, $p=0.34$) |
| *Miscelaneous* | | | | | | |
| Honow 2003 [32] | 500 mL or 1,000 mL apple juice from "master product" (Hamburger Warencenter, Hamburgh, Germany) vs. mineral water | 9 | Healthy female volunteers, compared with controls | 0.11 (500 mL daily intake) or 0.23 (1,000 mL daily intake) | 234 kcal (500 mL daily intake) or 468 kcal (1,000 mL daily intake) estimated | 21.2% increase (500 mL daily intake) $p<0.05$; 41.2% increase (1,000 mL daily intake); $p<0.01$ |
| Kessler 2002 [33] | 330 mL blackcurrant juice diluted with up to 420 mL water | 12 | Healthy volunteers, up to 750 mL diluted blackcurrant juice. Comparison vs. mineral water control phase | 49.5 mEq | 122 kcal | 25.1% increase; $p<0.01$ |
| – | 330 mL plum juice diluted with up to 420 mL water | 12 | Healthy volunteers, up to 750 mL diluted plum juice. Comparison vs. mineral water control phase | 0.69 mEq | 184 kcal | 2.1% increase; $p=$NS |

*NS* not significant

Group, Plano, TX, USA) diluted to 2 L with tap water significantly increased 24-h urine citrate excretion in patients with hypocitraturic calcium oxalate nephrolithiasis from a mean of 142–346 mg per day [3]. In their study, 11 of the 12 participants experienced increased urine citrate, while urine calcium excretion decreased and urine oxalate levels were unchanged. All subjects enrolled in the study completed a 1-week trial of homemade lemonade, and the cost of treatment was estimated by the authors to be US$ 2 per week. Aras et al. studied the effects of a solution of 60 mL of fresh-squeezed lemon juice diluted in 1 L of water, compared to drinking 1 L of water [19]. They found that urine citrate excretion in patients with hypocitraturic calcium nephrolithiasis increased 2.4-fold over baseline, compared with a 0.4-fold increase in controls, which was highly statistically significant, $p=0.001$ [19]. A single long-term retrospective study examined stone recurrence in 11 patients with hypocitraturic nephrolithiasis treated with the homemade lemonade described by Seltzer et al. The authors reported significant sustained increases in citraturia over baseline as well as a significant reduction in yearly stone formation from 1 to 0.13 stones per year over a 4-year period [26].

Despite these findings, several studies have shown little or no benefit of lemonade therapy. In a study of 21 patients, half of whom had hypocitraturia, Koff et al. found that potassium citrate increased urine citrate, but a homemade lemonade solution of 30 mL ReaLemon concentrate juice with three-fourths cup (177 mL) of water did not [25]. Odvina examined 14 volunteers (ten nonstone formers and four patients with a history of nephrolithiasis) and reported that a commercial lemonade (Minute Maid, 400 mL three times per day) failed to raise urine citrate [20]. Penniston et al. examined homemade lemonade therapy alone versus the combination of lemonade (same formula as used by Seltzer et al.) and potassium citrate. They reported that the combination therapy resulted in sustained elevation of urine citrate, but lemonade therapy alone did not [21].

In summary, while results are mixed regarding lemonade therapy, many believe it is a reasonable option for patients with nephrolithiasis and low urine citrate. In addition to possibly raising urine citrate, lemonade may be more palatable in large quantities than water for some patients, which may help them maintain higher urine volumes. One common approach is to recheck urine citrate levels after several months on lemonade therapy, and if it does not appear to be effective, to switch to pharmacological treatment such as potassium citrate.

## Lime Juice

A study of lime juice made from freeze-dried lime powder mixed with potassium in stone formers with hypocitraturia demonstrated significant increases in urine citrate (increase of 383 %) [27]. In this study, the manufacturing of the beverage included the freeze-drying of lime juice using commercial-grade equipment as well as the addition of pharmaceutical-grade potassium (details not specified) to the lime juice mixture. The results, therefore, are difficult to interpret in terms of the contribution of the lime juice alone versus the juice with added potassium to citraturia observed in these patients. da Cunha Baia et al. reported on transient changes in urine citrate after ingestion of 75 mL of lime juice diluted in 310 mL of water by measuring urine citrate at baseline and 2, 4, and 6 h after ingestion. Citraturia was noted to increase significantly over baseline at 2 and 4 h, but returned to baseline level by 6 h after ingestion. It is unclear how these findings are related to 24-h urine citrate excretion, which is the standard of measurement in the rest of the literature [22].

## Orange Juice

Despite lower overall citrate content than lemons, oranges contain citrate complexed with potassium (i.e., citrate as alkali), making orange juice a potentially attractive dietary source for raising urine citrate. Odvina performed a crossover study of 14 patients, examining the effects of commercial preparations of orange juice and lemonade (Minute Maid, Houston, TX, USA) on urinary citrate levels [20]. Urinary citrate excretion was significantly increased on orange juice therapy (mean increase of $\sim 500$ mg/day in urine citrate, $p < 0.05$) while no difference was observed with lemonade therapy (mean increase of $\sim 50$ mg/day citrate, $p = $ NS). Of note, the caloric content of orange juice resulted in an intake of 550 kcal of carbohydrate during the orange juice phase, which might have its own deleterious side effects by causing unwanted weight gain. Honow et al. in 2003 reported similar results, demonstrating a 36 % increase in urinary citrate over a mineral water placebo when orange juice was consumed, but at the cost of 448 kcal daily [32]. A similar study comparing the effect of 1.2 L of orange juice daily versus 60 mEq of potassium citrate daily in tablet form found that orange juice delivered an equivalent alkali load, an equivalent increase in urinary citrate but also increased urinary oxalate, which could be deleterious for calcium oxalate stone formers [28]. da Cunha Baia et al. also reported significant increases in citraturia over baseline for orange juice consumption at 2, 4, and 6 h after consumption, as well as an increase in urine pH at 4 h, which returned to baseline at 6 h [22]. Thus, despite the efficacy of orange juice in raising urine citrate, practitioners must take caution in using high volumes of orange juice on a chronic basis for citrate replacement, due to its high caloric content and potential to raise urine oxalate.

## Cranberry Juice

There is evidence that cranberry juice contains amounts of citrate similar to that of lemonade [39]. Several studies have been performed, with discordant results. One study, which examined 12 normal subjects and 12 calcium oxalate stone formers, demonstrated that a daily consumption of 1 L of cranberry juice (Ocean Spray) had no effect on urine citrate, but resulted in significantly increased urine calcium and oxalate [23]. Kessler et al. showed no effect on urinary citrate with ingestion of 330 mL of cranberry juice per day [33]. A study of 20 healthy male students randomized to drinking either 2 L of tap water daily or 500 mL of cranberry juice (Crystal Falls, Black Sheep Beverage Distributors, South Africa) with 1,500 mL of water demonstrated an increase in urinary citrate by 31 % ($p<0.001$) with the diluted cranberry juice [34]. Similar to orange juice, the high caloric content of cranberry juice may result in unwanted carbohydrate consumption with this type of therapy.

## Grapefruit Juice

Two studies have examined the effects of grapefruit juice on urine citrate excretion. Goldfarb and Asplin examined urine chemistries in healthy men and women who consumed 240 mL of grapefruit juice (Tropicana Products, Chicago, IL, USA) three times per day [35]. Urine citrate significantly increased by a mean of 85 mg per day ($p=0.01$) and urine oxalate increased by a mean of 10 mg per day ($p=0.001$). It is unclear what the net effect on stone risk is due to these observed increases in citrate and oxalate, but calcium oxalate supersaturation did not change. Honow et al. studied the effects of 500 or 1,000 mL of grapefruit juice administered daily to nine healthy female volunteers [32]. They found a 20.5 % increase in urinary citrate in the 500-mL group and a 47.6 % increase in the 1,000-mL group over baseline. This is associated with some caloric load intake (196.5 and 393 kcal/day, respectively). Urinary oxalate was not significantly increased. Epidemiologic studies on grapefruit juice have produced equivocal results. In 1996, Curhan et al. reported that consumption of grapefruit juice was associated with an increased risk of kidney stone formation (37 % for every 240-mL serving consumed daily), but an update of their cohort data nearly 17 years later failed to demonstrate a significant association between grapefruit juice consumption and stone risk [42, 43].

## Sports Drinks

Goodman et al. compared the effect of two citrus-based sports drinks, Performance (Shaklee Corp., Pleasanton, CA, USA) and Gatorade (Gatorade, Chicago, IL, USA) on 24-h urine composition in 19 nonstone formers. Subjects drank 946 mL (32 oz) of tap water daily for 3 days, and recorded diet history then consumed either Performance or Gatorade after a washout period. Performance significantly increased urine citrate excretion by 170 mg/day and urine pH by 0.31, but Gatorade did not change either parameter significantly. The quantity of Performance ingested during this study would result in a daily intake of 400 kcal. Thus, Performance appears to have significant effects on urine citrate, which may be similar in magnitude to those observed in some studies using homemade lemonade [36].

## Carbonated Beverages

A recent study reported the citrate as alkali content of commonly consumed diet sodas compared with that in homemade lemonade used by Seltzer et al. This demonstrated that several citrus-based sodas (Diet 7-up, Diet Sunkist Orange, Sierra Mist Free, Sprite Zero, Fresca, Diet Canada Dry, Diet Mountain Dew, and Fanta Zero Orange) contained greater amounts of citrate as alkali than lemonade [44]. The effects of water consumption, diet cola, and a grapefruit-based diet soda on 24-h urine citrate have been examined. In six volunteers, 24-h urine composition was studied after intake of Le Bleu water, caffeine-free Diet Coke, and Fresca in a crossover design. None of these beverages increased 24-h urine citrate, despite similar citrate content between Fresca and homemade lemonade [37]. A similar study in nine volunteers showed no effect of Diet Sunkist Orange soda on urinary citrate excretion at the volume consumed, 1,064 mL/day [38]. It remains unclear as to why these diet sodas (Fresca and Diet Sunkist) failed to raise urine citrate in a similar fashion to lemonade. It is possible that these studies were either underpowered in terms of subjects, or that the quantity of diet soda was too low to demonstrate a significant change in urine citrate. A caveat to recommending these beverages in addition to the lack of experimental evidence is that diet sodas, consumed in large quantities, may have other deleterious effects due to their acid, phosphorous, and artificial sweetener content.

Karagülle et al. studied two types of carbonated mineral water (commercially available in Germany) with concentrations of bicarbonate differing by an order of magnitude (99 mg/L vs. 2.67 mg/L) in patients with recurrent calcium stones. They reported significant increases in urine pH (baseline <6.3 to mean of 6.83 after treatment) as well as significant increases in urine citrate [24].

## Other Juices

In a single study of blackcurrants, 12 healthy subjects drank 330 mL of unsweetened blackcurrant juice diluted with 420 mL of water; it was observed that urinary citrate increased 25 % over baseline ($p<0.01$). Caloric intake for this beverage is estimated at 122 kcal/serving [33, 40]. Plum juice has a very low amount of citrate, at approximately 2 mEq/L. The same authors demonstrated no significant change in urinary citrate with daily ingestion of 330 mL of plum juice [33]. In addition, it has an unfavorable caloric profile, at over 500 kcal/L, making plum juice a less-promising therapy. In a single study, apple juice, though extremely low in citrate and providing little citrate load, increased urinary citrate by 21.2 % when 500 mL was consumed daily or 41.2 % when 1,000 mL was consumed daily by healthy volunteers. Caloric load was 234 kcal or 468 kcal, respectively.

## Epidemiologic Observations

Several epidemiologic cohort studies have been published on the topic of beverage use and the risk of kidney stones [16, 42, 45, 46]. The most recent study, published in 2013, was an update of earlier studies published in the 1990s. A prospective examination of cohorts of nearly 52,000 men, 122,000 younger women, and 116,000 older women, the following associations between beverage intake and kidney stone risk were reported: Kidney stone risk is increased with increasing consumption of sugar-sweetened colas and noncolas, artificially sweetened colas and noncolas, and fruit punch, while kidney stone risk was decreased with increasing consumption of caffeinated coffee, decaffeinated coffee, tea, wine, beer, and orange juice. Though previous studies from this group reported increasing stone risk with consumption of apple juice or grapefruit juice, this updated data analysis failed to show these associations [42]. As these are epidemiologic cohort studies, the effects of these various beverages on 24-h urine composition were not examined. A previously published study comparing stone formation among monozygotic and dizygotic twins reported a protective effect on stone risk for those who drank at least one cup of milk per day compared with those who did not consume milk [46].

## Selection of Appropriate Treatment

In our own practice for those with calcium stones and hypocitraturia, we review that potassium citrate is the gold standard therapy [13]. If patients are averse to pharmacotherapy, we use the lemonade formula for lemonade described originally by Seltzer et al. [3]. We also review lemonade therapy as an option for patients who have not undergone a complete metabolic workup but are interested in dietary advice on how to decrease the risk of stone recurrence. Our choice of lemonade is based on aforementioned data as well as the concern for high caloric intake associated with other beverages that are known to raise urine citrate. Patients are advised to drink the homemade lemonade daily and 24-h urine composition is then rechecked 3–4 months after the initiation of lemonade therapy. If lemonade is ineffective at raising urine citrate based on this 24-h urine collection, it is recommended that the patients change to potassium citrate for treatment of their hypocitraturia. We feel that it is also reasonable to review the option for lemonade therapy for first-time stone formers in whom a full metabolic evaluation is deferred until a possible future stone recurrence. For these patients, in addition to the typical recommendation of >2 L of fluid consumption per day [16], we review that the addition of either fresh-squeezed lemon juice or reconstituted lemon juice may be beneficial in terms of urine citrate excretion. We have particular concern about the recommendation of beverages with high caloric/carbohydrate content, with respect to both kidney-stone and weight-gain risks. If prescribed daily, many fruit juices and sweetened beverages could lead to weight gain; obesity and diabetes have each been shown in prospective studies to increase the risk of urolithiasis [47].

# Conclusion

Dietary therapy for low urine citrate is an area in which there is demonstrated patient interest. Studies and results are equivocal, and sometimes apparently contradictory. Although beverages have shown the potential to raise urine citrate (i.e., lemonade, orange juice, cranberry juice, limeade), no particular beverage has performed consistently enough to be adopted by the urologic and medical community at large. None of these beverages has been shown to reduce stone incidence or recurrence in a prospective trial. In addition, of the beverages that do increase urine citrate, only the lemonade reported by Seltzer et al. does not have associated unwanted caloric and carbohydrate intake. Future studies should be aimed at targeting beverages with the highest content of citrate as alkali, while also minimizing caloric intake for the patients on this type of therapy.

# References


1. Tracy CR, Pearle MS. Update on the medical management of stone disease. Curr Opin Urol. 2009 Mar;19(2):200–4.
2. Eisner BH, Sheth S, Dretler SP, Herrick B, Pais VM Jr. Abnormalities of 24-hour urine composition in first-time and recurrent stone-formers. Urology. 2012 Oct;80(4):776–9.
3. Seltzer MA, Low RK, McDonald M, Shami GS, Stoller ML. Dietary manipulation with lemonade to treat hypocitraturic calcium nephrolithiasis. J Urol. 1996 Sep;156(3):907–9.
4. Zuckerman JM, Assimos DG. Hypocitraturia: pathophysiology and medical management. Rev Urol. 2009 Summer;11(3):134–44.
5. Mossetti G, Vuotto P, Rendina D, Numis FG, Viceconti R, Giordano F, et al. Association between vitamin D receptor gene polymorphisms and tubular citrate handling in calcium nephrolithiasis. J Intern Med. 2003 Feb;253(2):194–200.
6. Eisner BH, Porten SP, Bechis SK, Stoller ML. The role of race in determining 24-hour urine composition in white and Asian/Pacific islander stone formers. J Urol. 2010 Apr;183(4):1407–11.
7. Pak CY, Fuller C, Sakhaee K, Preminger GM, Britton F. Long-term treatment of calcium nephrolithiasis with potassium citrate. J Urol. 1985 Jul;134(1):11–9.
8. Soygur T, Akbay A, Kupeli S. Effect of potassium citrate therapy on stone recurrence and residual fragments after shockwave lithotripsy in lower caliceal calcium oxalate urolithiasis: a randomized controlled trial. J Endourol. 2002 Apr;16(3):149–52.
9. Sarica K, Erturhan S, Yurtseven C, Yagci F. Effect of potassium citrate therapy on stone recurrence and regrowth after extracorporeal shockwave lithotripsy in children. J Endourol. 2006 Nov;20(11):875–9.
10. Singh SK, Agarwal MM, Sharma S. Medical therapy for calculus disease. BJU Int. 2011 Feb;107(3):356–68.
11. RxPriceQuotes . 2013 http://www.rxpricequotes.com/.
12. Drugstore.com, Inc. 2013. http://drugstore.com/.
13. Barcelo P, Wuhl O, Servitge E, Rousaud A, Pak CY. Randomized double-blind study of potassium citrate in idiopathic hypocitraturic calcium nephrolithiasis. J Urol. 1993 Dec;150(6):1761–4.
14. Tiselius HG. Patients' attitudes on how to deal with the risk of future stone recurrences. Urol Res. 2006 Aug;34(4):255–60.
15. Grampsas SA, Moore M, Chandhoke PS. 10-year experience with extracorporeal shockwave lithotripsy in the state of colorado. J Endourol. 2000 Nov;14(9):711–4.

16. Borghi L, Meschi T, Amato F, Briganti A, Novarini A, Giannini A. Urinary volume, water and recurrences in idiopathic calcium nephrolithiasis: a 5-year randomized prospective study. J Urol. 1996 Mar;155(3):839–43.
17. Curhan GC, Willett WC, Knight EL, Stampfer MJ. Dietary factors and the risk of incident kidney stones in younger women: nurses' health study II. Arch Intern Med. 2004 Apr 26;164(8):885–91.
18. Taylor EN, Stampfer MJ, Curhan GC. Dietary factors and the risk of incident kidney stones in men: new insights after 14 years of follow-up. J Am Soc Nephrol. 2004 Dec;15(12):3225–32.
19. Aras B, Kalfazade N, Tugcu V, Kemahli E, Ozbay B, Polat H, et al. Can lemon juice be an alternative to potassium citrate in the treatment of urinary calcium stones in patients with hypocitraturia? A prospective randomized study. Urol Res. 2008 Dec;36(6):313–7.
20. Odvina CV. Comparative value of orange juice versus lemonade in reducing stone-forming risk. Clin J Am Soc Nephrol. 2006 Nov;1(6):1269–74.
21. Penniston KL, Steele TH, Nakada SY. Lemonade therapy increases urinary citrate and urine volumes in patients with recurrent calcium oxalate stone formation. Urology. 2007 Nov;70(5):856–60.
22. Baia Lda C, Baxmann AC, Moreira SR, Holmes RP, Heilberg IP. Noncitrus alkaline fruit: a dietary alternative for the treatment of hypocitraturic stone formers. J Endourol. 2012 Sep;26(9):1221–6.
23. Gettman MT, Ogan K, Brinkley LJ, Adams-Huet B, Pak CY, Pearle MS. Effect of cranberry juice consumption on urinary stone risk factors. J Urol. 2005 Aug;174(2):590, 4; quiz 801.
24. Karagulle O, Smorag U, Candir F, Gundermann G, Jonas U, Becker AJ, et al. Clinical study on the effect of mineral waters containing bicarbonate on the risk of urinary stone formation in patients with multiple episodes of CaOx-urolithiasis. World J Urol. 2007 Jun;25(3):315–23.
25. Koff SG, Paquette EL, Cullen J, Gancarczyk KK, Tucciarone PR, Schenkman NS. Comparison between lemonade and potassium citrate and impact on urine pH and 24-hour urine parameters in patients with kidney stone formation. Urology. 2007 Jun;69(6):1013–6.
26. Kang DE, Sur RL, Haleblian GE, Fitzsimons NJ, Borawski KM, Preminger GM. Long-term lemonade based dietary manipulation in patients with hypocitraturic nephrolithiasis. J Urol. 2007 Apr;177(4):1358, 62; discussion 1362; quiz 1591.
27. Tosukhowong P, Yachantha C, Sasivongsbhakdi T, Ratchanon S, Chaisawasdi S, Boon-la C, et al. Citraturic, alkalinizing and antioxidative effects of limeade-based regimen in nephrolithiasis patients. Urol Res. 2008 Aug;36(3–4):149–55.
28. Wabner CL, Pak CY. Effect of orange juice consumption on urinary stone risk factors. J Urol. 1993 Jun;149(6):1405–8.
29. Taylor EN, Curhan GC. Dietary calcium from dairy and non-dairy sources and risk of symptomatic kidney stones. J Urol. 2013 Mar 24;190(4):1255–9.
30. Taylor EN, Fung TT, Curhan GC. DASH-style diet associates with reduced risk for kidney stones. J Am Soc Nephrol. 2009 Oct;20(10):2253–9.
31. Khan A, Housami F, Melotti R, Timoney A, Stickler D. Strategy to control catheter encrustation with citrated drinks: a randomized crossover study. J Urol. 2010 Apr;183(4):1390–4.
32. Honow R, Laube N, Schneider A, Kessler T, Hesse A. Influence of grapefruit-, orange- and apple-juice consumption on urinary variables and risk of crystallization. Br J Nutr. 2003 Aug;90(2):295–300.
33. Kessler T, Jansen B, Hesse A. Effect of blackcurrant-, cranberry- and plum juice consumption on risk factors associated with kidney stone formation. Eur J Clin Nutr. 2002 Oct;56(10):1020–3.
34. McHarg T, Rodgers A, Charlton K. Influence of cranberry juice on the urinary risk factors for calcium oxalate kidney stone formation. BJU Int. 2003 Nov;92(7):765–8.
35. Goldfarb DS, Asplin JR. Effect of grapefruit juice on urinary lithogenicity. J Urol. 2001 Jul;166(1):263–7.
36. Goodman JW, Asplin JR, Goldfarb DS. Effect of two sports drinks on urinary lithogenicity. Urol Res. 2009 Feb;37(1):41–6.

                                                      M. P. Kurtz and B. H. Eisner

37. Passman CM, Holmes RP, Knight J, Easter L, Pais V, Assimos DG. Effect of soda consumption on urinary stone risk parameters. J Endourol. 2009 Mar;23(3):347–50.
38. Sumorok NT, Asplin JR, Eisner BH, Stoller ML, Goldfarb DS. Effect of diet orange soda on urinary lithogenicity. Urol Res. 2012 Jun;40(3):237–41.
39. Haleblian GE, Leitao VA, Pierre SA, Robinson MR, Albala DM, Ribeiro AA, et al. Assessment of citrate concentrations in citrus fruit-based juices and beverages: implications for management of hypocitraturic nephrolithiasis. J Endourol. 2008 Jun;22(6):1359–66.
40. Yilmaz E, Batislam E, Basar M, Tuglu D, Erguder I. Citrate levels in fresh tomato juice: a possible dietary alternative to traditional citrate supplementation in stone-forming patients. Urology. 2008 Mar;71(3):379, 83; discussion 383–4.
41. Yilmaz E, Batislam E, Kacmaz M, Erguder I. Citrate, oxalate, sodium, and magnesium levels in fresh juices of three different types of tomatoes: evaluation in the light of the results of studies on orange and lemon juices. Int J Food Sci Nutr. 2010 Jan 29;61(4):339–45.
42. Ferraro PM, Taylor EN, Gambaro G, Curhan GC. Soda and other beverages and the risk of kidney stones. Clin J Am Soc Nephrol. 2013 May 15;8(8):1389–95.
43. Curhan GC, Willett WC, Rimm EB, Spiegelman D, Stampfer MJ. Prospective study of beverage use and the risk of kidney stones. Am J Epidemiol. 1996 Feb 1;143(3):240–7.
44. Eisner BH, Asplin JR, Goldfarb DS, Ahmad A, Stoller ML. Citrate, malate and alkali content in commonly consumed diet sodas: implications for nephrolithiasis treatment. J Urol. 2010 Jun;183(6):2419–23.
45. Curhan GC, Willett WC, Speizer FE, Stampfer MJ. Beverage use and risk for kidney stones in women. Ann Intern Med. 1998 Apr 1;128(7):534–40.
46. Goldfarb DS, Fischer ME, Keich Y, Goldberg J. A twin study of genetic and dietary influences on nephrolithiasis: a report from the vietnam era twin (VET) registry. Kidney Int. 2005 Mar;67(3):1053–61.
47. Taylor EN, Stampfer MJ, Curhan GC. Diabetes mellitus and the risk of nephrolithiasis. Kidney Int. 2005 Sep;68(3):1230–5.

# Chapter 5
# Bariatric Surgery and Stone Disease: Help or Hindrance?

**Gautam Jayram and Brian R. Matlaga**

## Introduction

As of 2012, over 150 million Americans are considered overweight, and over half of this population has a body mass index (BMI) $>30$ kg/m$^2$ [1]. Furthermore, total health care costs attributable to obesity are estimated to be 16–18% of all health care expenditures by 2030. Obese patients have a marked increase in their risk of type II diabetes, hypertension, sleep apnea, cardiovascular disease, and ultimately risk of early death [2]. Although not usually grouped with the others, nephrolithiasis represents an important condition significantly impacted by obesity. Epidemiological studies have suggested an association between obesity and kidney stones, and the coincidental increase in the prevalence of both conditions signify a potentially shared pathophysiology between the two [3–5].

Dietary changes, exercise programs, and pharmacologic approaches to weight loss are routinely implemented as an initial health improvement strategy. These therapies, however, suffer from inconsistent results, significant reaccumulation of lost weight, and high attrition rates [6, 7]. Consequently, bariatric surgery has become an increasingly popular weight loss intervention. Recent years have demonstrated a surge in the utilization of these procedures, as they have been shown to not only reliably produce weight loss, but also improve obesity-related comorbidities and reduce long-term mortality [8]. From a nephrolithiasis standpoint, bariatric surgery produces conflicting physiologic effects that are still being elucidated. Some of these effects, may increase the risk for kidney stone formation. Controversy exists as to the overall impact of weight loss surgery on the incidence, risk profile, and epidemiology of urinary stone disease, and consequently there has been increased academic interest in this subject. This chapter gives an overview of the effect bariatric surgery has on kidney stone disease and attempts to provide evidence-based answers to the controversies raised in the field.

B. R. Matlaga (✉) · G. Jayram
The Johns Hopkins Hospital, James Buchanan Brady Urological Institute,
600 North Wolfe Street, Park 221, Baltimore, MD 21287, USA
e-mail: bmatlaga@jhmi.edu

M. S. Pearl, S. Y. Nakada (eds.), *Practical Controversies in Medical Management of Stone Disease,* DOI 10.1007/978-1-4614-9575-8_5,
© Springer Science+Business Media New York 2014

## Obesity and Urolithiasis

Metabolic syndrome encompasses the pathophysiologic changes imparted by obesity that ultimately lead to an increased risk of cardiovascular disease. In one study, the prevalence of nephrolithiasis in individuals with metabolic syndrome was 9 % and shown to increase as the prevalence of the individual components of the syndrome increased as well [9]. A study of geographically restricted patients in Southern Italy demonstrated a twofold greater occurrence of objectively demonstrated nephrolithiasis in patients with metabolic syndrome than those without [10]. Several larger population-based studies have confirmed a direct, positive association between increasing BMI and the risk of kidney stone formation [3, 5]. Semins et al elaborated on these findings by demonstrating no appreciable increase in stone disease after a BMI of 30, suggesting a plateau effect in pathophysiologic mechanisms responsible for this phenomenon [11].

Multiple factors account for the increased risk of urinary stone disease in obese patients. In a study of morbidly obese patients scheduled for gastric bypass, 98 % had at least one risk factor for kidney stone formation and 80 % had three or more risk factors [12]. Increased intake of lithogenic substances, such as sugars, purine-rich foods, calcium, and oxalate is commonly seen in these patients. In addition, obesity and metabolic syndrome are commonly associated with insulin resistance (including type II diabetes mellitus), which alters renal handling of acids and decreases ammoniagenesis. The resulting increasingly acidified urinary load will promote the precipitation of uric acid and decrease the urinary excretion of citrate. The latter abnormality is of particular lithogenic concern, as citrate is known to be a potent inhibitor of kidney stone formation. Obese stone formers have also been shown to have excessive urinary excretion of sodium, calcium, and uric acid; their urinary pH, too, is decreased when compared to nonobese stone formers [13–15]. It has also been theorized that hypertension, a common part of the obesity-metabolic syndrome complex, further contributes to stone formation by altering renal handling of calcium and causing hypercalciuria [16]. Finally, obese patients are at increased risk for gouty diathesis, which may further promote uric acid stone formation [12, 17].

## Surgical Therapy for Weight Loss

Bariatric surgical procedures induce weight loss by altering the anatomy of the gastrointestinal tract to restrict the amount of food that can be eaten at one time and/or decrease the length of intestine through which food can be absorbed. Bariatric surgery has evolved significantly from its roots in the early 1970s, and the restrictive and malabsorptive operations currently performed represent major advances over earlier procedures which were marred by severe complications. Jejunoileal bypass was the first surgical procedure utilized for the treatment of obesity, and it required an extreme degree of malabsorption, in essence creating a surgical "short gut" with a long blind loop of bowel. This bypass technique ultimately became obsolete, due to a high incidence of complications, including hepatic failure, nephropathy, and renal stones, the latter thought to result from severe hyperoxaluria due to malabsorption [18, 19]. Consequently, the Food and Drug Administration requested a moratorium on the procedure in 1979, and the procedure was abandoned [20].

Contemporary bariatric procedures rely on more moderate alterations of gastrointestinal physiology, and typically function through caloric restriction, malabsorption, or both. Restrictive procedures such as gastric banding or sleeve gastrectomy limit food intake at any given time by decreasing the size of the gastric pouch [21]. Other procedures, such as biliopancreatic diversion (duodenal switch) and Roux-en-Y gastric bypass (RYGB), combine some level of gastric resection with variable amounts of intestinal bypass. Although the utilization of bariatric surgery appears to be slightly decreasing in recent years, there are still over 120,000 bariatric procedures performed in the USA annually, with RYGB being the most commonly performed operation [22].

## Impact of Bariatric Surgery on Urolithiasis

The new generation of bariatric procedures was intended to circumvent the disastrous metabolic complications of jejunoileal bypass. Specifically, these procedures claimed to induce less severe malabsorption than jejunoileal bypass, which may therefore result in a diminished risk of urinary stone disease. Multiple studies have been performed evaluating stone incidence and metabolic parameters in the modern bariatric surgical population. This next section describes the known evidence evaluating the effect of bariatric surgery on urine parameters and kidney stones.

### *Restrictive Procedures*

Gastric banding (GB) and sleeve gastrectomy (SG) are procedures that have gained popularity in the surgical treatment of obesity, now comprising 20–25 % of all weight-loss procedures [23]. These procedures have the advantage of avoiding intestinal bypass and theoretically imparting a minimal impact on metabolic stone disease. Semins et al. first described a significant decrease in the diagnosis of upper urinary tract calculi in over 200 patients undergoing GB compared with obese controls (1.5 vs. 6 %) with 2 years of follow-up from the National Inpatient Sample [24]. Less than 1 % of each cohort in the study ultimately required stone surgery. A study of 73 adolescents between the ages of 13 and 17 receiving laparoscopic gastric banding demonstrated a postoperative incidence of 1.4 % of symptomatic stone disease [25]. Chen et al. described the largest series to date of patients undergoing a restrictive bariatric procedure—417 without a previous stone history. The study found an incidence of 1.2 % (4/332) in the GB group and 1.18 % (1/85) in the SG group with 3.5 and 2 years of follow-up, respectively [26]. The majority of stone formers were asymptomatic, with only two of the five stone formers requiring surgery. Stone analysis from one patient revealed 100 % calcium oxalate monohydrate. These population-based studies suggest the lack of intestinal bypass does indeed confer a benefit on urinary stone formation. Furthermore, multiple studies have shown no demonstrable hyperoxaluria following both GB and SG, likely the protective clinical factor in minimizing stone disease [27, 28]. Clearly longer-term studies need to be performed to validate these findings. Based on existing clinical and urine chemistry data; however, modern restrictive bariatric procedures appear to succeed in decreasing the risk of urinary stone formation in obese patients.

## *Malabsorptive Procedures*

RYGB is currently the most common surgical intervention for morbid obesity, with >108,000 procedures performed annually [8]. Modern-day versions of this procedure bypass smaller lengths of intestine and hypothetically minimize the severity of metabolic complications. Specifically, RYGB works by surgically reducing the gastric reservoir as well as by bypassing a length of small intestine. As such, a lower caloric intake and reduced absorptive surface area have been shown to result in sustained weight loss, and improvements in hypertension, dyslipidemia, diabetes, and obstructive sleep apnea [29, 30]. As fat malabsorption is known to contribute to hyperoxaluria and urinary stone disease in the inflammatory bowel and short-gut population, there has been growing concern about the lithogenic effects of RYGB. Asplin et al. confirmed hyperoxaluria in the modern bariatric population (which included both RYGB and GB patients), demonstrating an adjusted mean urine oxalate excretion greater than double (83 mg/day) in post-surgical patients compared to stone formers not undergoing surgery (39 mg/day) and normal subjects (34 mg/day) [31]. In this study, patients treated with jejunoileal bypass had a mean urinary oxalate of 102 mg/day, considered to be a dangerous level of hyperoxaluria coincident with renal damage. Further studies have repeatedly confirmed hyperoxaluria in the RYGB cohort, and others have documented additional lithogenic effects on urine volume, urine citrate, and urine calcium [32–34]. Durrani provided the first clinical study demonstrating an increase in stone formation following RYGB. Following over 900 patients who underwent laparoscopic RYGB, the authors estimated an approximately 70 % increase in stone prevalence post-RYGB compared to expected rates derived from the National Health and Nutrition Examination Survey III [35]. Utilizing national claims data, Matlaga et al. reported the largest published study characterizing the impact of RYGB on clinically significant stone disease. This study evaluated over 4,600 patients matched with obese nonsurgical controls followed for over 3 years. The authors found RYGB to be associated with a higher rate of kidney stone diagnosis (7.7 vs. 4.6 %) as well as a higher rate of surgical treatment for a stone (3.3 vs. 0.9 %). Logistic regression and multivariate analysis indicated RYGB was a significant predictor of both stone diagnosis and undergoing a surgical procedure for stone disease [36]. Taken in sum, both laboratory and clinical data document an increased risk of stone disease following RYGB. These data must be interpreted with caution and await long-term validation; however, as RYGB does provide a sustained long-term benefit on overall health in the obese population that may outweigh its impact on stone disease.

## Managing Stone Risk Following Bariatric Surgery

Dietary counseling remains the foundation of stone prevention therapy for patients undergoing bariatric surgery. A target urine output of greater than 2 L per day is ideal; therefore, adequate fluid consumption is of particular importance as a stone prevention measure for patients undergoing bariatric surgery. It should be noted, though, that in the immediate postoperative period large, bolus-type fluid intake can be problematic; rather, such patients should administer a more continuous intake of small fluid volumes. This is primarily due to the restrictive component of many bariatric procedures which will limit boluses of food or water. Dietary recommendations for bariatric surgery patients include moderation of dietary oxalate and fat intake, and the recommended daily allowance of calcium (1,000–12,000 mg/day) to begin early postoperatively [37].

To better define the need for more specific dietary interventions for bariatric surgery patients who form kidney stones or who are at risk for kidney stone formation, more complete studies, such as a 24-h urine metabolic evaluation, are required. Dietary maneuvers based on the findings of such studies may include restricted sodium, animal protein, and oxalate intake. Rigorous oxalate restriction can be challenging; in some cases, over 50 % of daily excreted oxalate is derived from endogenous sources. Oxalate restriction can be frustrating for the patient, as most foods are poorly labeled for oxalate content. It should also be noted that sufficient calcium intake is necessary to prevent stone formation, and in certain cases, based on the results of a complete metabolic evaluation, calcium supplements can be employed as a means to increase oxalate elimination. A small study by Pang et al. demonstrated that a controlled metabolic diet (low oxalate, normal calcium, and moderate protein) decreased calcium oxalate supersaturation in patients post-bariatric surgery, but did not reduce hyperoxaluria [38]. The timing of calcium supplement administration is of importance; the calcium should be present in the intestinal lumen at the time of oxalate intake for proper and effective binding. Oral citrate supplementation can also be administered to increase urinary pH in the setting of particularly acidic urine, or for urinary citrate repletion in the setting of hypocitraturia. Undertaking these maneuvers may pose particular challenges to the bariatric surgery patient, though, which must be recognized. For example, patients with restrictive surgery must modify their eating habits to take small frequent meals to avoid dumping syndrome. Consequently, the use of oxalate-binding agents such as calcium supplements as well as increasing fluid intake can be difficult to comply with.

Novel therapeutic agents may hold some benefit for bariatric surgery patients who are at increased risk for stone formation. The oral administration of *Oxalobacter formigenes* or its oxalate-degrading enzymes for patients with hyperoxaluria may increase colonic metabolism of oxalate to prevent systemic absorption. In small series, the oral administration of *O. formigenes* reduced plasma oxalate and urinary oxalate excretions in those with primary hyperoxaluria [39, 40]. Although this therapeutic option certainly requires further investigation, it may ultimately have a role in managing stone risk among bariatric hyperoxaluric patients.

For patients who have undergone jejunoileal bypass and have severe, refractory side effects, including stone disease, reversal of bypass can be performed. Although surgical reversal will normalize urinary oxalate excretion, patients may continue to form stones and suffer from persistent hypocitraturia [41]. There may be a benefit to undertaking urinary pH manipulation with citrate administration in an effort to further reduce stone risk among such patients.

## Conclusion

The increased risk of stone disease induced by certain bariatric procedures is a significant health concern. However, this concern must be measured against the substantial overall health benefits of surgically induced weight loss. Preoperative counseling is required for all patients, but is of particular importance for those with a history of stone disease who, therefore, may be at increased risk for a stone following bariatric surgery. It is important to know which procedure is optimal for each patient, given the multiplicity of interventions available. To that end, future studies should better define the optimal procedure for patient subgroups. For example, are purely restrictive procedures safer for patients with a history of stone disease? Other important questions include whether additional measures of prevention or surveillance are warranted in these populations—and if so, what are optimal schedules and methods for surveillance? Is routine metabolic screening of bariatric patients warranted from a clinical or economic standpoint? Novel approaches for the management of enteric hyperoxaluria are also of importance, as it can be particularly challenging for patients to adhere to simple dietary restrictions. A better understanding of the mechanisms of hyperoxaluria in bariatric patients would also be welcome, as it may better inform the risk modification. Finally, an improved understanding of the causes and the natural course of hyperoxaluria will help improve prevention and treatment of stone disease in these patients.

## References


1. American Heart Association. Statistical Fact Sheet Update. http://www.heart.org/idc/groups/heart-public/@wcm/@sop/@smd/documents/downloadable/ucm_319588.pdf (June 10, 2013).
2. Roth J, Qiang X, Marban SL, Redelt H, Lowell BC. The obesity pandemic: where have we been and where are we going? Obes Res 2004;12:88.
3. Taylor EN, Stampfer MJ, Curhan GC. Obesity, weight gain, and the risk of kidney stones. JAMA. 2005;293:455.

4.  Stamatelou KK, Francis ME, Jones CA, Nyberg LM, Curhan GC. Time trends in reported prevalence of kidney stones in the United States, 1976–1994. Kidney Int. 2004;63:1817.

5.  Curhan GC Willett WC, Rimm EB, Speizer FE, Stampfer MJ. Body size and risk of kidney stones. J Am Soc Nephrol. 1998;9:1645.

6.  NIH Conference. Gastrointestinal surgery for severe obesity. Consensus development conference panel. Ann Intern Med. 1991;115:956.

7.  Glenny AM, O'Meara S, Melville A, Sheldon TA, Wilson C. The treatment and prevention of obesity: a systematic review of the literature. Int J Obes Relat Metab Disord. 1997;21:715–37.

8.  Santry HP, Gillen DL, Lauderdale DS. Trends in bariatric surgical procedures. JAMA. 2005;294:1909.

9.  West B, Luke A, Durzao-Arvizu RA, Cao G, Shoham D, Kramer H. Metabolic syndrome and self-reported history of kidney stones: the national health and nutrition examination survey (NHANES III) 1988–1994. Am J Kidney Dis. 2008;51:741–7.

10. Rendina D, Mossetti G, De Filippo G, Benvenuto D, Vivona CL, Imbroinise A, et al. Association between metabolic syndrome and nephrolithiasis in an inpatient population in southern Italy: role of gender, hypertension, and abdominal obesity. Nephrol Dial Transplant. 2009;24:900–6.

11. Semins MJ, Shore AD, Makary MA, Magnuson T, Johns R, Matlaga BR. The association of increasing body mass index and kidney stone disease. J Urol. 2010 Feb; 183(2):571–5.

12. Duffey BG, Pedro RN, Kriedberg C, Weiland D, Melquist J, Ikramuddin S, et al. Lithogenic risk factors in the morbidly obese population. J Urol. 2008;179:1401.

13. Maalouf NM, Sakhaee K, Parks JH, Coe FL, Adams-Huet B, Pak CY. Association of urinary pH with body weight in nephrolithiasis. Kidney Int. 2004;65:1422–5.

14. Taylor EN, Curhan GC. Body size and 24-hour urine composition. Am J Kidney Dis. 2006;48:905–15.

15. Abate N, Chandalia M, Cabo-Can AV Jr, et al. The metabolic syndrome and uric acid nephrolithiasis: novel features of renal resistance. Kidney Int 2004;65:386–92.

16. Cappuccio FP, Strazzullo P, Mancini M, Moe OW, Sakhaee K. Kidney stones and hypertension: an independent clinical association in a population based study. BMJ 1990;300:1234–6.

17. Ekeruo WO, Tan YH, Young MD, Dahm P, Maloney ME, Mathias BJ, et al. Metabolic risk factors and the impact of medical therapy on the management of nephrolithiasis in obese patients. J Urol. 2005;172:159.

18. Kirkpatrik JR. Jejunoileal bypass. A legacy of late complications. Arch Surg 1987;122:610–4.

19. Nelson Andersson H, Bosaeus I. Hyperoxaluria in malabsorptive states. Urol Int 1981;36:1–9.

20. Requarth JA, Burchard KW, Colacchio TA, Stukel TA, Mott LA, Greenberg ER, et al. Long-term morbidity following jejunoileal bypass. The continuing potential need for surgical reversal. Arch Surg. 1995;130:318.

21. Belachew M, Legrand M, Vincent V, Lismonde M, Le Docte N, Deschamps V. Laparoscopic adjustable gastric banding. World J Surg 1998;22:955.

22. Nguyen NT, Masoomi H, Magno CP, Nguyen XM, Laugenour K, Lane J. Trends in use of bariatric surgery, 2003–2008. J Am Coll Surg. 2011 Aug;213(2):261–6.

23. Hinojosa MW, Vareal JE, Parikh D, Smith BR, Nguyen XM, Nguyen NT. National trends in use and outcome of laparoscopic adjustable gastric banding. Surg Obes Relat Dis. 2009;5:150–155.

24. Semins MJ, Matlaga BR, Shore AD, Steele K, Magnuson T, Johns R, et al. The effect of gastric banding on kidney stone disease. Urology. 2009 Oct;74(4):746–9.

25. Nadler EP, Young HA, Ren CJ, Fielding GA. An update on 73 US obese pediatric patients treated with laparoscopic adjustable gastric banding: comorbidity resolution and compliance data. J Pediatr Surg. 2008 Jan; 43(1):141–6.

26. Chen T, Godebu E, Horgan S, Mirheydar HS, Sur RL. The effect of restrictive bariatric surgery on urolithiasis. J Endourol. 2013 Feb;27(2):242–4.

27. Semins MJ, Asplin JR, Steele K, Assimos DG, Lingeman JE, Donahue S, et al. The effect of restrictive bariatric surgery on urinary stone risk factors. Urology. 2010 Oct;76(4):826–9.

28. Penniston KL, Kaplon DM, Gould JC, Nakada SY. Gastric band placement for obesity is not associated with increased urinary risk of urolithiasis compared to bypass. J Urol. 2009 Nov;182(5):2340–6.
29. Buchwald H, Avidor Y, Braunwald E, Jensen MD, Pories W, Fahrbach K, et al. Bariatric surgery: a systematic review and meta-analysis. JAMA 2004;292:1724–37.
30. Patriti A, Facchiano E, Sanna A, Gullà N, Donini A. The enteroinsular axis and recovery from type 2 diabetes after bariatric surgery. Obes Surg 2004;14:840–8.
31. Asplin JR, Coe FL. Hyperoxaluria in kidney stone formers treated with modern bariatric surgery. J Urol. 2007 177:565–9.
32. Wu JN, Craig J, Chamie K, Ali MR, Low RK. Urolithiasis risk factors in the bariatric population undergoing gastric bypass surgery. Surg Obes Relat Dis. 2013 Jan-Feb;9(1)83–7.
33. Duffey BG, Alanee S, Pedro RN, Hinck B, Kriedberg C, Ikramuddin S, et al. Hyperoxaluria is a long-term consequence of Roux-en-Y gastric bypass: a 2-year prospective longitudinal study. J Am Coll Surg. 2010 Jul;211(1):8–15.
34. Maalouf NM, Tondapu P, Guth ES, Livingston EH, Sakhaee K. Hypocitraturia and hyperoxaluria after Roux-en-Y gastric bypass surgery. J Urol. 2010 Mar;183(3):1026–30.
35. Durrani O, Morrisroe S, Jackman S, Averch T. Analysis of stone disease in morbidly obese patients undergoing gastric bypass surgery. J Endourol. 2006 Oct; 20(10):749–52.
36. Matlaga BR, Shore AD, Magnuson JM, Clark JM, Johns R, Makary MA. Effect of gastric bypass surgery on kidney stone disease. J Urol. 2009 Jun;181(6):2573–7.
37. Furtado LC. Nutritional management after Roux-en-Y gastric bypass. Br J Nurs. 2010 Apr 8–21;19(7):428–36.
38. Pang R, Linnes MP, O'Conner HM, Li X, Bergstralh E, Lieske JC. Controlled metabolic diet reduces calcium oxalate supersaturation but not oxalate excretion after bariatric surgery. Urology. 2012 Aug;80(2):250–4.
39. Siva S, Barrack ER, Reddy GP, Thamilselvan V, Thamilselvan S, Menon M, et al. A critical analysis of the role of gut Oxalobacter formigenes in oxalate stone disease. BJU Int. 2009 Jan;103(1):18–21.
40. Siener R, Bangen U, Sidhu H, Hönow R, von Unruh G, Hesse A. The role of Oxalobacter formigenes colonization in calcium oxalate stone disease. Kidney Int. 2013 Jun;83(6):1144–9.
41. Dhar NB, Grundfest S, Jones JS, Streem SB. Jejunoileal bypass reversal: effect on renal function, metabolic parameters and stone formation. J Urol. 2005 Nov;174(5):1844–6.

# Chapter 6
# Protein Restriction and Stone Disease: Myth or Reality?

Sara L. Best

## Introduction

Dietary modification is a ubiquitous component of the modern management of nephrolithiasis. These recommendations are based on the long-existing knowledge that the characteristics of ingested food and drink are reflected in the byproducts of human metabolism, urine, and stool. Thus, manipulating potentially lithogenic risk factors by altering diet makes pathophysiologic sense. Indeed, a variety of investigations, often in nonstone-forming subjects, have demonstrated that alterations in diet can result in a change in urinary components such as calcium, sodium, etc., and yet other studies have proposed pathophysiologic explanations for these findings.

One dietary recommendation commonly made to stone formers is the restriction of dietary protein consumption. This recommendation is primarily based on observations from metabolic studies that show a variety of lithogenic changes associated with a dietary protein load, including a rise in urinary calcium and uric acid and a decrease in urinary citrate and pH. These effects are multifactorial and incompletely understood but are felt to relate to the acid and purine load associated with protein.

However, despite these seemingly "straightforward" effects of protein on urine parameters, epidemiological, observational, and randomized control studies have failed to convey a unanimous message regarding the impact of dietary protein manipulation on actual stone recurrence risk. This chapter will review the available literature on this topic.

S. L. Best (✉)
Department of Urology, University of Wisconsin School of Medicine and Public Health, 1685 Highland Ave, MFCB-3229, Madison, WI 53705, USA
e-mail: best@urology.wisc.edu

M. S. Pearle, S. Y. Nakada (eds.), *Practical Controversies in Medical Management of Stone Disease,* DOI 10.1007/978-1-4614-9575-8_6,
© Springer Science+Business Media New York 2014

                                                              

## Epidemiologic Studies

The notion of a relationship between protein consumption and stone risk has appeared in the literature for decades (Table 6.1). Several authors cite DA Andersen's 1973 essay, "Environmental Factors in the Aetiology of Urolithiasis," as some of the first epidemiologic evidence of a possible dietary protein link with upper tract stone formation [1]. In this essay, the author notes that while the incidence of bladder stones (particularly in children) appeared to decline with increasing affluence in developing countries, upper urinary tract stones became more common with industrialization. He reported a four times higher risk of nephrolithiasis in more affluent northwestern India compared to southeastern (23.6 vs. 5.9 admissions/10,000 inpatients), which he hypothesized might be related to a two times higher animal protein intake in the northwestern regions. Robertson and colleagues [2] proposed a similar hypothesis in 1979 after reviewing data from the UK that revealed a 45% rise in the number of annual inpatient discharges for urinary calculi between 1958 and 1969. The authors noted a rise in the expenditure on food and animal protein consumption during the same time period. While both papers are careful to note that other factors may certainly play a role, these and other early works led to other larger and more in-depth epidemiologic investigations into the role of dietary protein and lithogenesis.

Since these early reports, several long-term, population-based longitudinal studies designed to investigate links between health outcomes and diet have been established. Curhan and colleagues evaluated 45,619 men with no history of nephrolithiasis enrolled in the Health Professionals Follow-up Study (HPFS) [3]. The male participants, aged 40–75, provided health and dietary records (via food frequency questionnaires, FFQs) periodically over 4 years. Dietary intake of animal protein was found to be directly associated with an increased risk of stone formation. The relative risk of receiving a new diagnosis of nephrolithiasis was 1.33 in those men with the highest animal protein intake ($\geq 77$ g/d) compared to the lowest (50 g/d) (95% confidence interval (CI), 1.00–1.77).

In contrast, analysis of similar large population-based studies in women did not find as clear a correlation between stone risk and high dietary protein. In their 1997 paper reviewing the data from the Nurses Health Study I (NHS I), Curhan et al. [4] found no significant difference in protein consumption and incident stone risk over the 12-year course of the study ($p = 0.53$), but reported that if only the more recent data from 1986 to 1992 were analyzed, the relative risk of those women with the highest animal protein intake ($> 76$ g/d) was 1.36 compared to the lowest quintile ($< 42$ g/d) (0.99–1.86, $p \geq 0.05$). The authors comment that they felt the more detailed FFQs used in 1986 better captured accurate animal protein intake and may explain the difference. Similarly, Sorensen and coauthors [5] found no association between incident stone risk and dietary animal protein in the somewhat older cohort of women (aged 50–79) participating in Women's Health Initiative Observational Study. However, the Nurses' Health Study II (NHS II) reported a potential trend towards a *lower* stone risk for participants (all female) who consumed the *most*

**Table 6.1** Epidemiologic studies

| Study/year published | No. of participants | Name of study group | Participant characteristics | Follow-up period | Measurements used | Findings |
|---|---|---|---|---|---|---|
| Andersen (1973) [1] | NR | | Hospital stone admissions in India | NR | No. of upper tract stone admissions/10,000 patients, geographic economic development status differences | 4x ↑ risk of stones in more affluent Northwest (NW)  India compared to Southeast (SE) (23.6 vs. 5.9 admissions/10,000 inpatients), ascribed to 2x ↑ AP intake |
| Robertson (1979) [2] | Based on population of the UK 1958–1969 | | All patients in the UK discharged for "urinary calculi" | N/A | Report on Hospital Inpatient Enquiry (1958–1973) and Scottish Health Statistics (1962–1975), data on household consumption and expenditure on food from Annual Report on the National Food Survey Committee | 45 % ↑ in #annual inpatient discharges for urinary calculi between 1958 and 1969<br><br>Authors noted a ↑ in the expenditure on food and AP consumption during same time period |
| Curhan et al. (1993) [3] | 45,619 | HPFS | Men aged 40–75 | 4 years | Lifestyle/health questionnaires, FFQs | Quintile with highest animal protein intake (≥77 g/d) had ↑ risk of stones compared to lowest quintile (≤50 g/d) (relative risk (RR) 1.33, 95 % CI 1.00–1.77) |
| Curhan et al. (1997) [4] | 91,731 | NHS I | Female nurses aged 30–55 | 12 years | Lifestyle/health questionnaires, FFQs | No difference in incident stone risk in 12-year follow-up ($p$ =0.53)<br>1986–1992 data only: Quintile with highest AP intake ( >76 g/d) had ↑ risk of stones compared to lowest quintile (<42 g/d) RR 1.36 (0.99–1.86)[a] |
| Curhan et al. (2004) [10] | 96,245 | NHS II | Female nurses aged 25–42 | 8 years | Lifestyle/health questionnaires, FFQs | Quintile with highest AP intake (≥78 g/d) had ↓ risk of stones compared to lowest quintile (≤51 g/d) RR 0.84 (0.68–1.04) |

**Table 6.1** (continued)

| Study/year published | No. of participants | Name of study group | Participant characteristics | Follow-up period | Measurements used | Findings |
| --- | --- | --- | --- | --- | --- | --- |
| Goldfarb et al. (2005) [32] | 6,782 (3,391 responding twin pairs) | Vietnam Era Twin (VET) Registry | Male–male twin pairs born 1939–1955, both twins having served in the military from 1965 to 1975 | N/A | Health questionnaire with single question re: lifetime h/o nephrolithiasis Brief FFQs | Univariate analysis: Consumers of the highest levels of meat and fish less likely to report a history of stones than those who consumed the lowest amount of meat and fish (OR = 0.5, 95 % CI 0.3–0.9) This difference not significant on multivariate analysis |
| Sorenson et al. (2012) [5] | 78,293 | Women's Health Initiative Observational Study | Postmenopausal women age 50–79 with no history of nephrolithiasis at entry | Mean 8 yr | FFQs, health questionnaires | Dietary AP not associated with incident kidney stone risk on multivariate analysis |
| Mandel et al. (2013) [15] | 2,561 | HPFS NHS I NHS II | Men aged 40–75 Women 25–42 Women 30–55 | N/A | FF/health questionnaires, two 24-h urine collections | No difference in nondairy AP intake between SFs and non-SFs in any cohort Nondairy animal protein intake was associated with lower Ucit (per 10 g/d, −20 mg/d; 95 % CI [−29 to −11], $p < 0.001$) |

*AP* animal protein, *FFQ* food frequency questionnaire, *N/A* not applicable, *NR* not reported, *SF* stone former

[a] Authors hypothesize that shorter 1980 diet questionnaires may not have captured protein intake as well as longer 1986 questionnaire and that this may explain the difference

animal protein ($\geq 78$ g/d) compared to the lowest quintile of consumption ($\leq 51$ g/d) (RR 0.84, 95% CI 0.68–1.04, $p=0.05$ for multivariate analysis). These studies, conducted in similar fashions though in different populations, highlight that even from a population-based perspective, the relationship between protein consumption and stone risk is likely multifactorial and incompletely understood. Whether gender or age-based differences in protein metabolism explain these differences, or other unaccounted-for influences explain the varying relationship between dietary protein and stones remains to be determined.

## The Effect of Dietary Protein on Urinary Risk Factors for Stone Formation

In an effort to better understand its relationship to stone formation, many researchers have investigated the influence of protein consumption on urine parameters linked to lithogenesis. Pathophysiologic studies have suggested a number of potentially lithogenic changes associated with a protein load. Protein consumption confers an acid load largely related to amino-acid metabolism. Animal protein, typically rich in purines and sulfur-containing amino acids, may have an even greater effect on acid–base status. The acid load may explain the decreased urine pH and citrate levels often seen with protein consumption. Purine metabolism has been cited as a source of uricosuria, and there are a number of both traditional and emerging theories on the calciuria seen with protein loading. The next few sections of this chapter will review both the case control studies linking dietary protein to changes in urinary chemistries as well as the data surrounding several controversies relating to the mechanisms of protein metabolism.

### *Case Control Studies*

In addition to the findings of the large epidemiologic studies described previously, researchers have identified potentially lithogenic dietary risk factors by comparing detailed dietary histories from both stone formers and individuals with no history of nephrolithiasis (Table 6.2). While Robertson et al. [6] reported that male stone formers had diets containing more total and animal protein than their healthy counterparts, Griffith et al. [7] and Fellström et al. [8] found no difference in total protein consumption between the two groups. Trinchieri and colleagues found that stone-forming and healthy women had similar levels of protein consumption, but this differed from their findings in men, where male stone formers had higher intake of calories, total and animal protein, calcium, and fiber [9]. Together with the mixed findings of larger epidemiologic studies [3–5, 10] with study populations of different genders, these investigations suggest potential gender-based differences in protein metabolism.

**Table 6.2** Case control studies of comparing the ambient diets of stone formers and controls with no history of stone disease

| Study/year published | No. of participants | Measurements used | Reported findings |
| --- | --- | --- | --- |
| Trinchieri et al. (1991) [9] | 146 controls<br>68 men, 77 women<br>103 recurrent SFs<br>65 men, 38 women | 24-h dietary record and 24-h urine collection | Women: no difference in protein consumption<br>Men: SFs had $\uparrow$ intake of calories, total and animal protein, calcium, and fiber |
| Robertson et al. (1979) [6] | 85 male calcium SFs<br>22 men controls | "Dietary histories" | Recurrent SFs had significantly $\uparrow$ baseline intakes of total protein than normal controls, nearly entirely attributable to greater intake of flesh protein |
| Griffith et al. (1981) [7] | 51 SFs<br>51 case-matched controls (urology inpatients admitted for nonstones) | Interview obtained a "full dietary history of an average weekly intake" | No difference in total protein intake between SFs and controls |
| Fellström et al. (1989) [8] | 20 recurrent calcium SFs<br>15 men, 5 women<br>20 controls (non-SF friends selected by each case) | 4-day food record and dietary history obtained by dietician | No statistically significant difference in purine or total protein intake between SFs and controls |
| Coe et al. (1976) [25] | Ten hyperuricosuric CaOx SFs<br>Five case-matched non-SF controls | Ambient diet determined via food records | SFs had $\uparrow$ purine intake than controls despite over-all similar calories per day (259 vs. 155 mg/day, $p<0.01$) |
| Brockis et al. (1982) [33] | 30 vegetarians<br>30 nonvegetarians<br>(all non-SFs)<br>15 men, 15 women in each | "Diet analysis" and 24-h urine collection | Only difference was $\uparrow$ Uua in nonvegetarians ($p<0.001$)<br>Uca directly associated with total protein intake ($p<0.05$) but not with specifically either animal or vegetable protein |

*CaOx* calcium oxalate, *SF* stone former, *Uca* urinary calcium, *Uox* urinary oxalate, *Uua* urinary uric acid

Investigators have sought to better characterize the effects of protein consumption on 24-h urine parameters through case control studies comparing urine tests before and after short-term prescribed diets containing varying protein loads. The details and results of these studies, some in stone patients and some in healthy people, appear in Table 6.3. Robertson and colleagues conducted two small studies varying dietary animal protein in healthy individuals [6]. In the first part of the study, participants underwent daily 24-h urines while consuming a diet containing 55 g/d of animal protein for 3 days, at which point the diet was augmented with 34 g/d of tuna. The second part of the study had three phases of decreasing dietary protein while keeping dietary calcium constant. In both studies, increased dietary animal protein was associated with a rise in urinary calcium and uric acid. Giannini et al. noted similar findings in their investigation of 18 hypercalciuric stone formers when they applied a 15-day dietary protein restriction: notably a normalization of urinary calcium values (375–259 mg/d, normal 108–300 mg/d, $p < 0.001$) and a significant reduction in urinary uric acid (521–420 mg/d, normal 250–745 mg/d, $p < 0.005$) [11]. They also reported the protein restriction was associated with a lower urinary oxalate and higher citrate levels.

Several studies investigated the metabolic impact of various popular "dietary regimens". Seiner and coworkers compared a typical animal protein-rich "Western" diet, a balanced omnivorous diet, and an ovo-lacto vegetarian diet and found a stepwise decrease in urinary uric acid (657 to 493 to 433 mg/day, $p < 0.001$) and increase in urine pH (5.95 to 6.51 and 6.80, $p < 0.001$) [12]. Breslau et al. also looked at several meat-restricted diets by conducting a randomized crossover study with three isocaloric arms matched in total protein, calcium, sodium, and phosphorus but with varying protein sources [13]. They reported that the animal protein-rich diet resulted in highest urinary uric acid, calcium, sulfate, and net acid excretion and lowest urinary citrate, oxalate, and pH, followed by the ovo-vegetarian, then strict vegetarian diets. Reddy and coauthors evaluated the impact of the popular "Atkins' style" diet, which emphasizes consumption of protein while restricting carbohydrates [14]. The Atkins' diets resulted in a significant rise in urinary calcium ($p < 0.0001$) and a drop in urine pH and citrate levels ($p = 0.0004$ and 0.004, respectively) after 7 days, compared to participants' ambient diets.

In 2013, Mandel et al. reported that their investigation of 2,561 participants from NHS I and II and HPFS who completed 24-h urine collections revealed that non-dairy animal protein intake was associated with lower urinary citrate excretion (per 10 g/d, −20 mg/d; 95 % CI (−29 to −11), $p < 0.001$) [15]. Dairy and vegetable protein intakes, on the other hand, were not correlated to citrate excretion.

Since much of the medical management of stone disease is predicated on modifying 24-h urine abnormalities, these studies make a compelling case for an increased lithogenic risk with a high protein diet. However, it is important to note that these are short-term studies and a longer exposure might allow induction of potentially compensatory hormone or enzyme pathways that could alter risk. Also, these well-controlled study diets may not be reflective of the normal home diets of many stone formers. Finally, 24-h urine findings may not directly correlate with an increased stone recurrence risk.

**Table 6.3** Case control studies of protein-related dietary interventions using 24-h urine values as endpoints

| Study/year published | No. of participants | Intervention performed | Measurements used | Reported findings |
|---|---|---|---|---|
| *Protein interventions* | | | | |
| Giannini et al. (1999) [11] | Ten male and eight female hypercalciuric SFs | 15-day 0.8 mg/kg/d of dietary protein (mean reduction of 32 g/d). (dietary Ca kept constant 15 days prior and throughout study period) | 24-h urines before and after diet intervention | Protein restriction normalized UCa (375–259 mg/d, normal 108–300 mg/d, $p < 0.001$) Uua ↓ from 521 to 420 mg/d, normal 108–300 mg/d, $p < 0.005$ Uox ↓ from 53 to 9 mg/d, normal 22–40 mg/d, $p < 0.01$) Ucit ↑ from 657 to 1,024 mmol/d (normal 500–1,036 mg/d, $p < 0.025$) |
| Siener et al. (2003) [12] | Ten healthy men (non-SF) | Four arms 1. 14-day "ambient" diet (but instructed to avoid organ meats and seafood) 2. 5-day Western Diet: high energy, alcohol and protein content (95 g/d) and a fluid intake of 1.5 L/d, 24 g/d fiber 3. 5-day Omnivorous Diet: 65 g protein/d, 2.5 L/d fluids, 28 g/d fiber 4. 5-day Lacto-ovo Vegetarian Diet: 65 g/d protein, 2.5 L/d fluids, 52 g/d fiber | Daily 24-h urines during intervention phases | Omnivorous and vegetarian diets had ↑ urine pH and volume and ↓ Uua than Western diet |
| Robertson et al. (1979) [6] | 1. Six non-SF men 2. Ten men and four women (all non-SF) | Two arms 1. Days 1–3: 55 g/d AP Days 4–12: 55 g/d AP+34 g/d of tuna 2. Days 1–4: 92 g/d AP Days 5–8: 48 g/d AP Days 9–12: 1 g/d AP (Ca kept constant) | Daily 24-h urines | 1. Adding 34 g/d tuna resulted in 23 % ↑ Uca, 24 % ↑ Uox, 48 % ↑ Uua 2. Decreasing dietary AP intake led to significant ↓ Uca, Uox, and Uua (actual values not given) |

**Table 6.3** (continued)

| Study/year published | No. of participants | Intervention performed | Measurements used | Reported findings |
|---|---|---|---|---|
| Fellstrom et al. (1983) [34] | Eight recurrent SFs | Days 1–14: low AP diet<br>Days 15–28: high AP diet | 24-h urines at the end of each phase | High AP diet resulted in<br>90 % ↑ in Uua ($p<0.001$)<br>34 % ↑ in UCa ($p<0.02$)<br>28 % drop in Ucit ($<0.001$)<br>↓ in pH 0.9 units[a] |
| Rotily et al. (2000) [35] | 96 idiopathic calcium SFs | *Three arms*<br>1. $n=34$, low AP (both meat and dairy) diet ($<10\%$ of calories)<br>2. $n=31$, high fiber diet (target $>25$ g/d<br>3. $n=31$, control group to continue ambient diet[b] | FFQs and 24-h urines at baseline and 4 months | Low AP arm had ↓ Uurea, Usulfate, Ucit. No change in Uca or Uox<br>Hypercalciuric pts on low AP diet had greater ↓ in Uca, 8.7–7.4 mmol/d, $p=0.08$<br>At 4 months, pts on HFD had lower urine output 2.2 down to 1.7 L/d, $p=0.002$). No other differences in urinary parameters |
| Breslau et al. (1988) [13] | 15 non-SFs | *Three arms*<br>1. Animal protein (meat and dairy)<br>2. Soy-based+eggs (ovo-vegetarian protein)<br>3. Soy/vegetarian (no eggs)[c] | 24-h urines on each of the last 4 days of each phase | Animal protein diet resulted in highest Uua, Uca, Usulf, and NAE and lowest Ucit, Uox, and pH, followed by the ovo-vegetarian then vegetarian diets |
| Reddy et al. (2002) [14] | Ten overweight non-SFs | *Three arms*<br>1. Ambient diet (mean 91 g/d protein)<br>2. High-protein (164 g/d), low-carbohydrate ("Atkins' induction") diet<br>3. Less restricted high-protein (170 g/d), low-carbohydrate ("Atkins' maintenance") diet | 24-h urines on each of the last 2 days of each phase | Urine pH and citrate were lower on both Atkins' style diets than ambient diets ($p=0.0004$ and 0.004)<br>Increased but nonsignificant rises in Uua seen on Atkins' phases<br>Uca significantly higher in both Atkins' phases ($p<0.0001$) |
| *Purine interventions* | | | | |
| Coe et al. (1976) [25] | Ten hyperuricosuric CaOx stone formers<br>Five case-matched non-SF controls | Two arms<br>Dietary purine loading via meat<br>3 days: 4 mg/kg<br>3 days: 6 mg/kg | 24-h urine measurement of urate on the third day of each phase | Linear relationship between purine consumption and urate excretion in both patients and controls |

**Table 6.3** (continued)

| Study/year published | No. of participants | Intervention performed | Measurements used | Reported findings |
|---|---|---|---|---|
| Pak et al. (1978) [24] | 11 male hyperuricosuric CaOx stone formers; Three male hyperuricosuric and hypercalciuric CaOx SF | 1. 12-day purine-restricted diet (9 pts) supplemented with 3 g/day of RNA during the last 6 days<br>2. Same study design repeated on eight patients with patients taking 300 mg/d of allopurinol | 24-h urines on Days 4–6 and 10–12 | 1. Urinary uric acid levels normalized during purine restriction and doubled during purine loading phase<br>2. Patients had no hyperuricosuria even on high purine diet while on allopurinol |
| Tracy et al. (2014) [26] | 15 non-SFs | Three-arm randomized crossover study, each phase 7 days<br>1. Beef<br>2. Chicken<br>3. Fish[d] | Serum chemistries and 24-h urines on the last 2 days of each phase | Serum uric acid elevated ($>6.0$ mg/dL) in all three phases of study<br>Beef diet was associated with lower uric acid values than either fish or chicken (6.5 vs. 7.0 and 7.3 mg/dL, $p=0.011$ and $p=0.001$)<br>Uua levels elevated ($>600$ mg/day) in all three phases of the study<br>Fish diet was associated ↑ Uua than either beef or chicken (712 vs. 638 and 641 mg/d, $p=0.003$ and 0.04)<br>No significant differences in urinary pH, sulfate, calcium, citrate, oxalate, or sodium were noted |

*AP* animal protein, *CaOx* calcium oxalate, *SF* stone former, *Uca* urinary calcium, *Ucit* urinary citrate, *Uox* urinary oxalate, *Uua* urinary uric acid

[a] all compared to low AP diet

[b] all three arms advised to maintain high water intake

[c] all three arms isocaloric, total protein 75 mg/d, constant Ca, Na, and P

[d] matched for calories, protein, Na, and Ca, and indexed to body weight

## Hypercalciuria and Protein Consumption

One of the links between stone formation and dietary protein consumption has been the observation that a dietary protein load can induce hypercalciuria, a known risk factor for nephrolithiasis. Studies estimate this correlation to be quantifiable as a 1-mg rise in 24-h urinary calcium for every 1 g increase in dietary protein [16, 17].

While this link between dietary protein and urinary calcium is well accepted and is one of the reasons for generalized recommendations for stone formers to restrict protein intake, the causative nature of this observation remains controversial.

Traditionally, the hypercalciuric response to a protein load was attributed to an increase in endogenous acid production ("acid ash"), particularly in animal-based foods rich in sulfur-containing amino acids, whose metabolism generates sulfate. This theory proposes that the acid load generated by a protein-rich diet results in mobilization of calcium and alkali from the skeletal system (the "bone buffer"). The increased filtered load of calcium then results in a rise in urinary calcium [18, 19].

More recently, however, some investigators have proposed that the calciuric effect of protein may not be strictly related to acid load. For example, Maalouf and colleagues [20] found that by administering twice-daily potassium citrate to a group of healthy volunteers, they could neutralize the acid load imparted by a high-protein diet, but it did not eliminate a rise in urinary calcium. Alkalinization did, however, correct the increase in supersaturation indices of calcium oxalate (CaOx) and uric acid associated with a high protein diet. They concluded that, at least in the short term, acid load alone does not appear to entirely account for the calciuric effect of protein.

In a series of publications, Kerstetter and colleagues have reported their investigations into the mechanism of the calciuric effect of protein that suggest alternative physiologic explanations [17, 21, 22]. They have used dual stable calcium isotopes to investigate the response to variations in dietary protein in healthy individuals. They reported that, rather than a protein load resulting in spilling of calcium in the urine directly from bone breakdown as proposed in the traditional theory, dietary protein appears to increase gastrointestinal absorption of calcium and actually decreases the proportion of urine calcium originating from the skeleton [21]. They and other authors have proposed that this mechanism is mediated by hormones involved in calcium homeostasis in the body, parathyroid hormone (PTH) [17, 23], and insulin-like growth factors (IGF)-1 [23]. Studies by Kerstetter et al. and Cao et al. found that a low protein diet results in secondary hyperparathyroidism, which may account for the hypercalciuria. Additionally, a high-protein diet also stimulated levels of IGF-1, a potent stimulator of bone formation, which may counteract the bone breakdown associated with an acid load [23].

## Role of Purines

Purines are organic compounds involved in many important biologic processes and include adenine, uracil, and guanine, which are important components of deoxy-

**Table 6.4** Purine content of selected foods. (Adapted with permission from [36], Copyright 1988, with permission from Elsevier)

|                    | Purine content (mg/100 g) |
|--------------------|---------------------------|
| Liver              | 286                       |
| Beef               | 90–125                    |
| Poultry            | 131                       |
| Pork               | 120                       |
| Fish, canned       | 206                       |
| Halibut/cod/haddock| 125                       |
| Mushrooms          | 47                        |
| Bread, white       | 12                        |

and ribonucleic acids (DNA and RNA), and other biomolecules such as ATP, cAMP, etc. Animal protein typically has a higher purine content than most vegetable-based foods and is thought to comprise the primary source of exogenous purine (Table 6.4). While most other mammals metabolize ingested purines to allantoin via the enzyme uricase, humans lack this enzyme and thus the end product of human purine metabolism is the less-soluble uric acid. Consequently, a purine load may lead to transient hyperuricemia and resultant hyperuricosuria. This relationship is why several studies have honed in on animal protein rather than total protein as a specific dietary risk factor.

Investigators have worked to delve further into the relative contribution of purine load to the lithogenic risk of dietary protein consumption since, as already discussed, protein also results in an acid load that is only partially purine related (see Table 6.3). To help control for this, Pak and colleagues enrolled hyperuricosuric male CaOx stone formers in a metabolic study aiming to carefully control purine consumption [24]. Nine participants were placed on a purine-restricted diet for 12 days that was supplemented with 3 g/d of RNA on Days 7–12. They found that 24-h urinary uric acid normalized during purine restriction in these male stone formers who were hyperuricosuric on their baseline home diets. They also reported that the urinary uric acid levels doubled during the purine-loading phase. Eight patients participated in a secondary study with the same study design but took allopurinol 300 mg/d, and this eliminated the hyperuricosuria seen during the purine-loading phase.

Coe and colleagues obtained baseline dietary information as well as serum and urine uric acid data on a group of ten hyperuricosuric CaOx stone formers and compared them to five normal controls [25]. They found that the stone-forming cohort had a significantly higher purine intake than controls despite overall similar calories per day (259 vs. 155 mg/day, $p < 0.01$) and that the majority of this intake could be ascribed to consumption of steak, poultry, and roast beef. Each participant then went through two 3-day purine-loading phases of 4 and 6 mg/kg of purine, mainly from meat, and the investigators reported a linear increase in urate excretion in both patients and controls.

Tracy and coauthors further studied the role of purine content in their three-phase, randomized crossover metabolic study comparing three types of animal protein (beef, chicken, fish) [26]. As shown in Table 6.4, fish often contains more purine per gram of protein than either red meat or poultry. Participants consumed each standard metabolic diet (total protein intake matched in each phase, 1.4 g/kg/d) for 1 week and serum and urine chemistries were obtained on the last 2 days of each phase. The estimated mean dietary purine content of each phase was lowest for chicken (268 mg/day), followed by beef (302 mg/day) and fish (471 mg/day). Serum uric acid levels were elevated (>6.0 mg/dL) in all three phases of study, although the beef phase was associated with lower uric acid values than either fish or chicken. Urinary uric acid levels also exceeded the normal range (>600 mg/day) for all three phases, but the fish diet was associated with statistically significantly higher levels of urinary uric acid than either beef or chicken. No significant differences in urinary pH, sulfate, calcium, citrate, oxalate, or sodium were noted. Saturation indices and relative saturation ratios, measures of stone propensity, were also calculated and, interestingly, were highest in the beef diet compared to the fish or chicken diets. The authors concluded that stone formers should be advised to limit their intake of all animal flesh.

From these studies and others, we can conclude there is a direct relationship between oral purine consumption and urinary uric acid levels. However, in his review of purine metabolism, Zöllner points out that the absorption and metabolism of the many different purines varies greatly (RNA is better absorbed than DNA, for example), and this may explain variations in urinary uric acid excretion even in isopurinic diets [27].

## Dietary Protein and Stone Recurrence Risk

While the urinary changes found after a protein load appear lithogenic, it does not necessarily follow that dietary protein consumption can be manipulated to reduce stone recurrence. Indeed, while the case control studies using 24-h urine values as outcomes are fairly homogeneous (see Table 6.3), randomized dietary studies have failed to show a definitive link between protein restriction and reduced stone risk.

To date, only three randomized, multiyear studies manipulating dietary protein to assess its impact on stone recurrence have appeared in the literature (Table 6.5). Hiatt and colleagues randomized 99 single-episode CaOx stone formers with a recent negative abdominal X-ray (KUB) to either a control diet or a high-fiber, low-animal-flesh diet (total protein target: 56–64 g/d) [28]. Both groups were advised to drink six to eight glasses of liquid and consume two servings of dairy daily. Participants were followed for a mean of 3.4 years with FFQs, 24-h urines, and KUBs for stone recurrence. The authors reported that the low-protein/high-fiber group had a *higher* relative risk of stone formation than the control group (24 vs. 4 %, relative risk (RR) 5.6, 95 % CI 1.2–26.1). However, they noted poor compliance with the dietary recommendations in the low-animal-protein/high-fiber group. Importantly and contrary to expectations, only the controls experienced a statistically significant decline in protein consumption as assessed by FFQs. This finding, likely explained by the intervention group having a much lower baseline protein consumption (85 vs. 104 g), makes the results of this study difficult to interpret.

**Table 6.5** Case control studies with protein-related dietary interventions using stone recurrence as an endpoint

| Study/year published | No. of participants | Characteristics of participants | Interventional performed | Follow-up period | Measurements used | Findings |
|---|---|---|---|---|---|---|
| Hiatt et al. (1996) [28] | 99 (78 after 21% lost to follow-up) | Single CaOx stone recent negative KUB, aged 20–60 | 1. Control<br>2. Intervention: decrease intake of animal flesh and high purine foods (dairy permitted) (total protein target 56–64 g/d), increase fiber and fruits/vegetables[a] | Up to 4.5 years (mean 3.4 years) | FFQs<br>24-h urines<br>KUBs<br>Stone recurrence defined as: stone passage or surgically removed, new stone on KUB | Patients on the restricted protein diet had ↑ RR of stone formation (24 vs. 4%, RR 5.6, 95% CI 1.2–26.1)<br>Baseline fluid intake 38% greater in controls<br>Poor compliance with low protein diet<br>Intervention group had much lower baseline protein consumption (85 vs. 104 g)<br>Only controls experienced a statistically significant decline in protein consumption |
| Borghi et al. (2002) [29] | 120 (103 after 14% dropout rate) | Men with recurrent CaOx stones and hypercalciuria | 1. $n=60$, normal Ca, low AP (52 g/d), low Na (50 mmol/d)<br>2. $n=60$, low calcium diet (10 mmol/d) | 60 months | 24-h urines<br>KUBs<br>Renal US<br>Stone recurrence defined as: symptomatic renal stone or new stone on imaging | Both groups experienced normalization of Uca levels<br>\|Low Ca diet had ↑ Uox (33.1–39.0 mg/d) compared to a ↓ in the normal Ca diet (37.0–29.0 mg/d) $p<0.001$<br>Normal Ca diet had a ↓ risk of stone recurrence (20 vs. 38%, RR 0.49, 95% CI 0.24–0.98, $p=0.04$) |

**Table 6.5** (continued)

| Study/year published | No. of participants | Characteristics of participants | Interventional performed | Follow-up period | Measurements used | Findings |
|---|---|---|---|---|---|---|
| Dussol et al. (2008) [30] | 175 (73 after 59% dropout rate) | Idiopathic calcium SFs, aged 18–70 | 1. $n=23$, low AP (both meat and dairy) diet (<13% of calories)<br>2. $n=27$, high fiber diet (target >25 g/d increase)<br>3. $n=23$, control group to continue ambient diet[b] | 4 years | FFQs 24-h urines "radiologic" studies and US yearly stone recurrence defined as: symptomatic stone or new stone or >50% ↑ size on imaging | No difference in stone recurrence amongst three arms Only 24-h urine parameter seen to change was ↓ Usulf in low AP diet (4.3–3.2 mmol/d, $p<0.01$) |

*AP* animal protein, *Ca* calcium, *CaOx* calcium oxalate, *FFQ* food frequency questionnaire, *SF* stone former, *Uca* urinary calcium, *Uox* urinary oxalate, *US* ultrasound, *Usulf* urinary sulfate

[a] both groups to eat two servings of dairy/day or take 500 mg Ca carbonate/day and drink 6–8 glasses liquid daily

[b] all three arms advised to maintain high water intake

In 2002, Borghi et al. conducted a 5-year randomized study in 120 hypercalciuric male CaOx stone formers [29]. Half the participants were instructed to follow a low-calcium diet (400 mg/d) while the other half were permitted normal calcium intake (1,200 mg/d) but advised to restrict animal protein and sodium consumption (52 g/d and 1,130 mg/d, respectively). Urinary calcium normalized in both groups of previously hypercalciuric men, but those following the normal-calcium/low-sodium/low-protein diet had a lower risk of stone recurrence than those restricting dietary calcium (20 vs. 38%, RR 0.49, 95% CI 0.24–0.98, $p=0.04$). However, because several dietary variables were manipulated in this study (sodium, calcium, and protein), the individual effect of animal protein cannot be assessed.

Both of these studies recommended multiple dietary changes and did not look exclusively at the effect of dietary protein restriction. In an effort to specifically evaluate protein independently, Dussol and colleagues designed a randomized study with three arms: a low-animal-protein diet (both meat and dairy), a high-fiber diet, and a control group to continue their ambient diet [30]. A total of 175 idiopathic calcium stone formers were randomized, though only 73 patients (41%) completed the study. Participants were followed with FFQs, 24-h urines, and yearly "radiological" and ultrasound studies for 4 years. The authors reported that no differences in stone recurrence rates were found amongst the three arms.

What explains the conflicting findings of these three studies, one of which found a higher relative risk with animal protein restriction, one a lower risk, and the third, no effect? A limitation of these studies is the significant dropout rate experienced by each (14–59%, Table 6.5). While not unexpected over the course of a multiyear trial such as these studies, these dropouts limited the evaluable data for these investigators. Additionally, the severity of recurrence risk likely differed between studies. Hiatt et al., for example, included only first-time stone formers, while the Borghi study only enrolled recurrent stone formers with hypercalciuria. It may be that only certain subpopulations of stone formers benefit from protein restriction. Finally, participant compliance with the dietary recommendations was notably poor. In the Hiatt study, for example, the intervention group failed to achieve any significant drop in their protein consumption despite counseling to do so, whereas, interestingly, the control group in this study *did* reduce their dietary protein over the time course of the study (possibly related to the control group's much greater baseline protein consumption, 104 vs. 85 g/d). Dussol and colleagues also noted that the animal protein restriction arm in their study failed to meet the recommended protein restriction target of <13% calories/day. While lack of compliance creates an inevitable problem for studies seeking to study the impact of an intervention, their findings likely mirror the "real world" challenges facing clinicians and patients: namely, that long-term lifestyle changes are often difficult to make.

## Limitations of the Literature

As reviewed in this chapter, there exists conflicting data on which to base recommendations for stone formers regarding dietary protein. As is often the case when there is a lack of consensus, this is largely due to limitations of the existing literature. Most of the studies relating to dietary protein and stone formers are short-term metabolic investigations using serum and urine parameters as endpoints, rather than long-term studies using stone recurrence as an endpoint. Additionally, many of these metabolic studies were conducted in nonstone-forming patients, who may metabolize protein and other dietary components differently. Finally, translating diet-associated differences in urine variables into clinically significant stone recurrence effects carries its own limitations.

In their meta-analysis of randomized controlled trials (RCTs) of dietary interventions to reduce stone recurrence, Fink and coauthors [31] noted a paucity of trials evaluating the independent effect of single dietary changes (i.e., protein restriction alone), as well as poor adverse event reporting. One of the reasons investigators likely design RCTs in this fashion is that these studies are expensive and time consuming, so applying multiple interventions as opposed to individual variables may be more efficient. It also, however, reflects a reality in dietary therapy: nutrients are not consumed as individual elements but instead as components of whole foods. A person may eat beef lasagna, not just "protein" and thus efforts to alter one's diet may have further impact on lithogenic risk than just the protein component alone. For example, Dussol and colleagues noted that they suspected their study participants were supplementing their diet with additional high-fiber, high-oxalate fruits and vegetables when they were instructed to reduce their animal protein intake [30]. Thus, studying and identifying "stone-friendly" foods rather than individual nutrients may prove more useful to clinicians and stone formers in the future.

## Conclusion

While dietary protein restriction has been a traditional component of medical management for stone formers, the evidence for this recommendation is mixed. Short-term metabolic studies of the impact of a protein load on urine chemistries show largely consistent lithogenic urinary effects, but the clinical RCTs do not show a definitive reduction in stone formation from dietary protein restriction. The existing literature has significant limitations, in part, because in the "real world" nutrients including protein are consumed as whole foods whose other components may also affect lithogenic risk. Future studies may help clarify these risks and help identify strategies to manipulate dietary protein in a way that reduces stone recurrence.

# References


1. Andersen D. Environmental factors in the aetiology of urolithiasis. Proceedings of the International Symposium on Renal Stone Research, 130–134. Editors D.L Cifuentes-, A. Rapado, and A. Hodgkinson. Karger, Basel. 1972.
2. Robertson WG, Peacock M, Hodgkinson A. Dietary changes and the incidence of urinary calculi in the U.K. between 1958 and 1976. J Chronic Dis. 1979;32(6):469–76.
3. Curhan GC, Willett WC, Rimm EB, Stampfer MJ. A prospective study of dietary calcium and other nutrients and the risk of symptomatic kidney stones. N Engl J Med. 1993 Mar 25;328(12):833–8. (Research Support, Non-U.S. Gov't Research Support, U.S. Gov't, P.H.S.).
4. Curhan GC, Willett WC, Speizer FE, Spiegelman D, Stampfer MJ. Comparison of dietary calcium with supplemental calcium and other nutrients as factors affecting the risk for kidney stones in women. Ann Intern Med. 1997 Apr 1;126(7):497–504. (Comparative Study Research Support, U.S. Gov't, P.H.S.).
5. Sorensen MD, Kahn AJ, Reiner AP, Tseng TY, Shikany JM, Wallace RB, et al. Impact of nutritional factors on incident kidney stone formation: a report from the WHI OS. J Urol. 2012 May;187(5):1645–9. (Research Support, N.I.H., Extramural Research Support, U.S. Gov't, Non-P.H.S.).
6. Robertson WG, Peacock M, Heyburn PJ, Hanes FA, Rutherford A, Clementson E, et al. Should recurrent calcium oxalate stone formers become vegetarians? Br J Urol. 1979 Dec;51(6):427–31.
7. Griffith HM, O'Shea B, Kevany JP, McCormick JS. A control study of dietary factors in renal stone formation. Br J Urol. 1981 Oct;53(5):416–20. (Comparative Study Research Support, Non-U.S. Gov't).
8. Fellstrom B, Danielson BG, Karlstrom B, Lithell H, Ljunghall S, Vessby B. Dietary habits in renal stone patients compared with healthy subjects. Br J Urol. 1989 Jun;63(6):575–80. (Research Support, Non-U.S. Gov't).
9. Trinchieri A, Mandressi A, Luongo P, Longo G, Pisani E. The influence of diet on urinary risk factors for stones in healthy subjects and idiopathic renal calcium stone formers. Br J Urol. 1991 Mar;67(3):230–6.
10. Curhan GC, Willett WC, Knight EL, Stampfer MJ. Dietary factors and the risk of incident kidney stones in younger women: Nurses' Health Study II. Arch Intern Med. 2004 Apr 26;164(8):885–91. (Research Support, U.S. Gov't, P.H.S.).
11. Giannini S, Nobile M, Sartori L, Dalle Carbonare L, Ciuffreda M, Corro P, et al. Acute effects of moderate dietary protein restriction in patients with idiopathic hypercalciuria and calcium nephrolithiasis. Am J Clin Nutr. 1999 Feb;69(2):267–71.
12. Siener R, Hesse A. The effect of a vegetarian and different omnivorous diets on urinary risk factors for uric acid stone formation. Eur J Nutr. 2003 Dec;42(6):332–7. (Clinical Trial Randomized Controlled Trial Research Support, Non-U.S. Gov't).
13. Breslau NA, Brinkley L, Hill KD, Pak CY. Relationship of animal protein-rich diet to kidney stone formation and calcium metabolism. J Clin Endocrinol Metab. 1988 Jan;66(1):140–6. (Comparative Study Research Support, U.S. Gov't, Non-P.H.S. Research Support, U.S. Gov't, P.H.S.).
14. Reddy ST, Wang CY, Sakhaee K, Brinkley L, Pak CY. Effect of low-carbohydrate high-protein diets on acid-base balance, stone-forming propensity, and calcium metabolism. Am J Kidney Dis. 2002 Aug;40(2):265–74. (Comparative Study Research Support, U.S. Gov't, P.H.S.).
15. Mandel EI, Taylor EN, Curhan GC. Dietary and lifestyle factors and medical conditions associated with urinary citrate excretion. Clin J Am Soc Nephrol. 2013 Feb 28;8(6):901–8.
16. Ginty F. Dietary protein and bone health. Proc Nutr Soc. 2003 Nov;62(4):867–76. (Review).
17. Kerstetter JE, O'Brien KO, Insogna KL. Low protein intake: the impact on calcium and bone homeostasis in humans. J Nutr. 2003 Mar;133(3):855S–61S. (Research Support, Non-U.S. Gov't Research Support, U.S. Gov't, Non-P.H.S. Research Support, U.S. Gov't, P.H.S. Review).

18. Barzel US, Massey LK. Excess dietary protein can adversely affect bone. J Nutr. 1998 Jun;128(6):1051–3. (Review).
19. Remer T. Influence of diet on acid-base balance. Semin Dial. 2000 Jul-Aug;13(4):221–6. (Review).
20. Maalouf NM, Moe OW, Adams-Huet B, Sakhaee K. Hypercalciuria associated with high dietary protein intake is not due to acid load. J Clin Endocrinol Metab. 2011 Dec;96(12):3733–40. (Clinical Trial Research Support, N.I.H., Extramural).
21. Kerstetter JE, O'Brien KO, Caseria DM, Wall DE, Insogna KL. The impact of dietary protein on calcium absorption and kinetic measures of bone turnover in women. J Clin Endocrinol Metab. 2005 Jan;90(1):26–31. (Research Support, Non-U.S. Gov't Research Support, U.S. Gov't, P.H.S.).
22. Kerstetter JE, O'Brien KO, Insogna KL. Dietary protein affects intestinal calcium absorption. Am J Clin Nutr. 1998 Oct;68(4):859–65. (Clinical Trial Randomized Controlled Trial Research Support, Non-U.S. Gov't Research Support, U.S. Gov't, Non-P.H.S. Research Support, U.S. Gov't, P.H.S.).
23. Cao JJ, Johnson LK, Hunt JR. A diet high in meat protein and potential renal acid load increases fractional calcium absorption and urinary calcium excretion without affecting markers of bone resorption or formation in postmenopausal women. J Nutr. 2011 Mar;141(3):391–7. (Clinical Trial Randomized Controlled Trial Research Support, Non-U.S. Gov't Research Support, U.S. Gov't, Non-P.H.S.).
24. Pak CY, Barilla DE, Holt K, Brinkley L, Tolentino R, Zerwekh JE. Effect of oral purine load and allopurinol on the crystallization of calcium salts in urine of patients with hyperuricosuric calcium urolithiasis. Am J Med. 1978 Oct;65(4):593–9. (Research Support, U.S. Gov't, P.H.S.).
25. Coe FL, Moran E, Kavalich AG. The contribution of dietary purine over-consumption to hyperpuricosuria in calcium oxalate stone formers. J Chronic Dis. 1976 Dec;29(12):793–800. (Research Support, U.S. Gov't, P.H.S.).
26. Tracy CR, Best SL, Bagrodia A, Poindexter JR, Adams-Huet B, Sakhaee K, et al. Animal protein and the risk of kidney stones: a comparative metabolic study of animal protein sources. J Urol. 2014; In press.
27. Zollner N. Purine and pyrimidine metabolism. Proc Nutr Soc. 1982 Sep;41(3):329–42. (Review).
28. Hiatt RA, Ettinger B, Caan B, Quesenberry CP, Duncan D, Citron JT. Randomized controlled trial of a low animal protein, high fiber diet in the prevention of recurrent calcium oxalate kidney stones. Am J Epidemiol. 1996 Jul 1;144(1):25–33.
29. Borghi L, Schianchi T, Meschi T, Guerra A, Allegri F, Maggiore U, et al. Comparison of two diets for the prevention of recurrent stones in idiopathic hypercalciuria. N Engl J Med. 2002 Jan 10;346(2):77–84.
30. Dussol B, Iovanna C, Rotily M, Morange S, Leonetti F, Dupuy P, et al. A randomized trial of low-animal-protein or high-fiber diets for secondary prevention of calcium nephrolithiasis. Nephron Clin Pract. 2008;110(3):c185–94. (Randomized Controlled Trial).
31. Fink HA, Akornor JW, Garimella PS, MacDonald R, Cutting A, Rutks IR, et al. Diet, fluid, or supplements for secondary prevention of nephrolithiasis: a systematic review and meta-analysis of randomized trials. Eur Urol. 2009 Jul;56(1):72–80. (Meta-Analysis Research Support, N.I.H., Extramural Research Support, Non-U.S. Gov't Research Support, U.S. Gov't, Non-P.H.S. Review).
32. Goldfarb DS, Fischer ME, Keich Y, Goldberg J. A twin study of genetic and dietary influences on nephrolithiasis: a report from the Vietnam Era Twin (VET) Registry. Kidney Int. 2005 Mar;67(3):1053–61. (Research Support, Non-U.S. Gov't Research Support, U.S. Gov't, Non-P.H.S. Twin Study).
33. Brockis JG, Levitt AJ, Cruthers SM. The effects of vegetable and animal protein diets on calcium, urate and oxalate excretion. Br j urol. 1982 Dec;54(6):590–3. (Comparative Study Research Support, Non-U.S. Gov't).

34. Fellstrom B, Danielson BG, Karlstrom B, Lithell H, Ljunghall S, Vessby B. The influence of a high dietary intake of purine-rich animal protein on urinary urate excretion and supersaturation in renal stone disease. Clin Sci (Lond). 1983 Apr;64(4):399–405. (Clinical Trial Controlled Clinical Trial Research Support, Non-U.S. Gov't).
35. Rotily M, Leonetti F, Iovanna C, Berthezene P, Dupuy P, Vazi A, et al. Effects of low animal protein or high-fiber diets on urine composition in calcium nephrolithiasis. Kidney Int. 2000 Mar;57(3):1115–23. (Clinical Trial Randomized Controlled Trial).
36. Brule D, Sarwar D, Savoie L. Purine content of selected Canadian food products. J Food Com Anal. 1988;1(2):130–8.

# Chapter 7
# Uric Acid Nephrolithiasis: Uric Acid or Urine pH?

Khashayar Sakhaee

## Introduction

There is diversity in the prevalence of uric acid nephrolithiasis in the world [1]. However, due to obesity and type 2 diabetes mellitus, it has been demonstrated that uric acid stones are more frequent in type 2 diabetic stone formers than non-diabetic stone formers [2, 3]. Furthermore, a higher prevalence of uric acid stones has been disclosed in obese stone formers. Greater body mass index (BMI) and type 2 diabetes have been found to be independent risk factors for uric acid stone development [4–6] (Fig. 7.1). Given the worldwide epidemics of obesity and type 2 diabetes, uric acid stones have emerged as a high burden on many nations.

## Epidemiology

There are worldwide variations in uric acid stone prevalence. The highest prevalence is reported in the Middle East and a few European countries. Uric acid stones comprise 8–10 % of all kidney stones in the United States. Moreover, the prevalence of uric acid nephrolithiasis and gout is significantly higher among the U.S. Hmong immigrant population [7, 8]. A high prevalence of the features of metabolic syndrome is commonly associated with uric acid nephrolithiasis in Western societies as well as Hmong populations born in the U.S. [2, 9, 10]. Thus, interplay between genetic and environmental factors play an important role in high incidence of uric acid prevalence. It was first established that stone formers with type 2 diabetes mellitus have uric acid stones as the main stone constituent more frequently than non-diabetic stone formers [11]. This greater prevalence among type 2 diabetic stone formers and obese subjects has since been confirmed by several investigators

K. Sakhaee (✉)
Charles and Jane Pak Center for Mineral Metabolism and Clinical Research,
University of Texas Soutwestern Medical Center, 5161 Harry Hines Blvd.,
Dallas, TX, 75390-8885, USA
e-mail: khashayar.sakhaee@utsouthwestern.edu

M. S. Pearl, S. Y. Nakada (eds.), *Practical Controversies in Medical Management
of Stone Disease,* DOI 10.1007/978-1-4614-9575-8_7,
© Springer Science+Business Media New York 2014

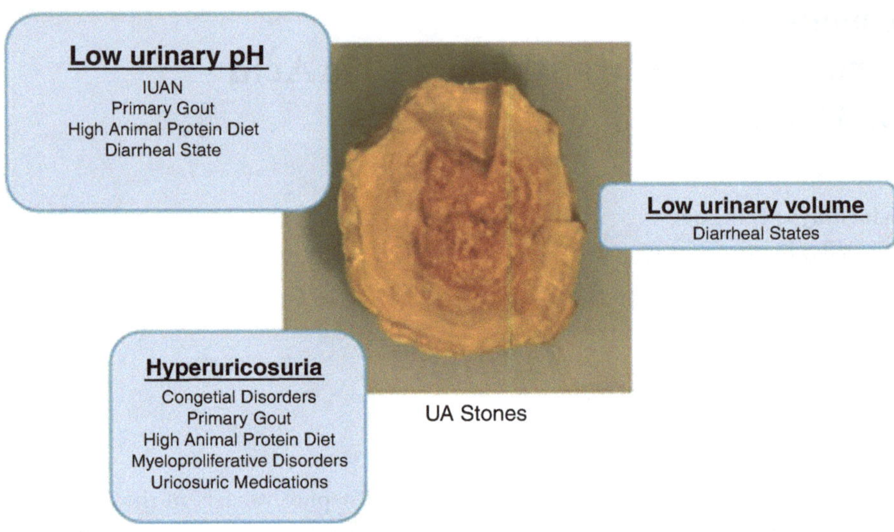



**Fig. 7.1** Pathophysiologic mechanisms and etiologic causes of uric acid nephrolithiasis

[7, 12]. Moreover, it was shown that greater BMI and type 2 diabetes are independent risk factors for uric acid nephrolithiasis [8].

## Physicochemical Characteristics of Uric Acid

In higher primates and humans, uric acid is produced as an end product of purine metabolism. This is then followed by metabolism of the hepatic enzyme uricase to the more soluble allantoin, which is then excreted into the urine [13]. However, humans and higher primates lack uricase; therefore, due to their lack of uric acid metabolism they display significantly higher urinary and serum concentration than other mammals [14]. This physiochemical principle plays an important clinical role in the management of patients with uric acid nephrolithiasis. Under normal circumstances, urinary uric acid solubility is limited to 96 mg/L. Since urinary uric acid excretion in humans varies between 600 and 800 mg/day, this high level of urinary uric acid exceeds the limit of solubility and poses a higher risk for uric acid precipitation and uric acid stone development [15, 16]. Thus, urinary pH plays a principal role in uric acid solubility of the urinary environment. Uric acid is a weak organic acid (pKa=5.5) [17, 18]. Given that abnormally low urine pH ($\leq$5.5) is the principal etiologic factor in the development of uric acid stones, it is obvious that in such urinary environments, urine is susceptible to supersaturation with respect to highly insoluble undissociated uric acid and thereby poses a higher risk of uric acid stone development [15, 19].

In earlier studies, patients with primary gout were shown to develop mixed uric acid and calcium stones [20]. However, until recently the underlying physicochemical and metabolic characteristics for calcium oxalate stone formation in patients with uric acid stones were not fully elucidated. In a retrospective study of 62 patients with pure uric acid stones and 101 patients with mixed uric acid and calcium oxalate stones, it was found that calcium oxalate stones may form in some patients with uric acid stones due to significantly increased urinary excretion of calcium and significantly lowered excretion of urinary citrate [21]. This observation, though retrospective and requiring further prospective investigation, may have therapeutic implications, since mixed uric acid and calcium oxalate stone patients can be treated with both thiazide and non-thiazide diuretics to lower urinary calcium excretion. Combined with optimal potassium alkali, this treatment has the potential to avoid highly alkaline urine above the pKa of phosphate (approximately 6.7) and lower the risk of calcium phosphate stone formation. While it does not negate the effect of rising urinary citrate, it aids in the inhibition of calcium oxalate and calcium phosphate agglomeration and crystal growth, respectively [22].

## Pathophysiological Mechanisms for the Development of Uric Acid Nephrolithiasis

The three important pathophysiologic mechanisms for development of uric acid stone formations are low urine volume, elevated urinary uric acid, and abnormally low urinary pH (Fig. 7.2). An unduly urinary acidity is the most prominent determinant in uric acid crystallization. Low urinary volume contributes to uric acid stone formation due to supersaturation of the urinary environment with undissociated uric acid. However, this may occur infrequently and is encountered only in patients with chronic diarrhea and excessive sweating due to strenuous physical exercise [23, 24]. Excessive purine ingestion may lead to hyperuricosuria, but generally patients with uric acid stones without dietary indiscretion are normouricosuric [15]. However, hyperuricosuria could be detected in rare genetic disorders that may lead to uric acid stone formation. Most distinctly, this abnormality was detected during childhood and manifested by an increased burden of kidney stones, renal impairment, and gout [25]. Furthermore, a specific genetic disorder characterized by mutations of uric acid transporter, URAT1, has been known to present with hyperuricosuria, high risk for uric acid stones, and characteristically with exercise-induced acute renal failure associated with hyperuricemia [26, 27].

However, urinary pH has been shown to be the most prevalent physiologic abnormality in patients with idiopathic uric acid nephrolithiasis and normouricosuria [15]. There are shared characteristics among obese stone formers and type 2 diabetic populations without kidney stones including hypertension, obesity, hypertriglyceridemia, hyperuricemia, and glucose intolerance [9, 28, 29]. Previous studies have shown that an impaired renal ammonium excretion, increased net acid excretion, or a combination of the two will result in overly acidic urine [9, 15]. These derangements were shown under both ad lib and fixed metabolic diets.

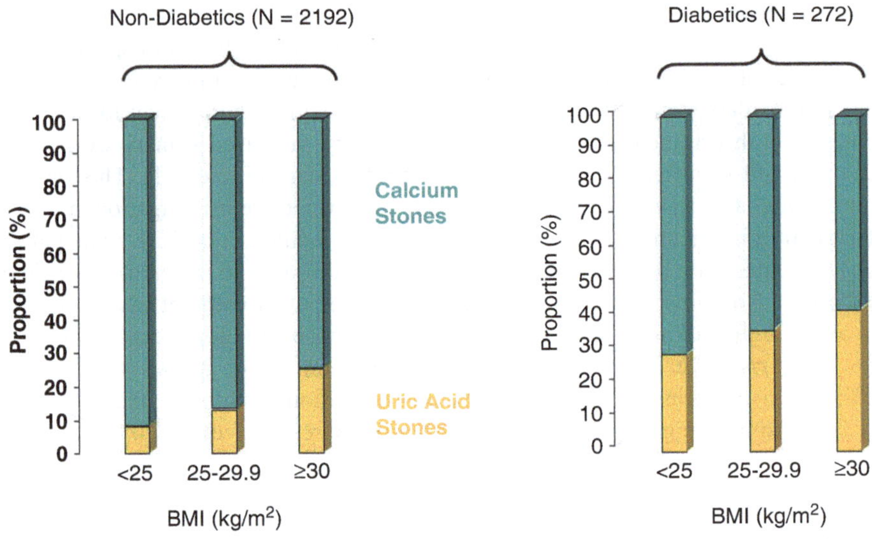



**Fig. 7.2** Distribution of stone type with respect to BMI and diabetes status. (Adapted from [6])

In normal circumstances, an acid–base balance is maintained tightly with the ability of the kidney to produce a high capacity buffer, ammonia (pKa = 9.2), which efficiently buffers most of the hydrogen secreted while the remaining protons are neutralized by numerous buffers collectively termed as "titratable acids." This tight mechanism will sustain normal urinary pH; however, the effective ammonium excretion in idiopathic uric acid nephrolithiasis subjects will cause the main urinary buffer to be titratable acid with a lower pKa than ammonia. Therefore, the acid–base equilibrium will be maintained, though at a low urinary pH. Thus, an acidic urinary pH provides an environment highly susceptible to uric acid precipitation and increases the risk of uric acid stone formation. Moreover, it has been demonstrated that a second mechanism may also be responsible for the unduly urine acidity in this population. Under a fixed metabolic diet and in a steady state, the urinary net acid excretion was found to be higher in uric acid stone formers and also in type 2 diabetic subjects without stones compared to normal subjects under the same dietary environment [13]. The nature and the site of increased putative organic anions have not yet been fully elucidated.

## Basic and Clinical Implications

In one study conducted under a fixed metabolic diet, comprising of 29 patients with isolated uric acid stones and/or mixed uric acid and calcium oxalate stones, 24 h urinary uric acid excretion ranged from 379 to 553 mg/day compared with normal subject levels of 498 mg/day [15]. This study also showed significantly lower urinary

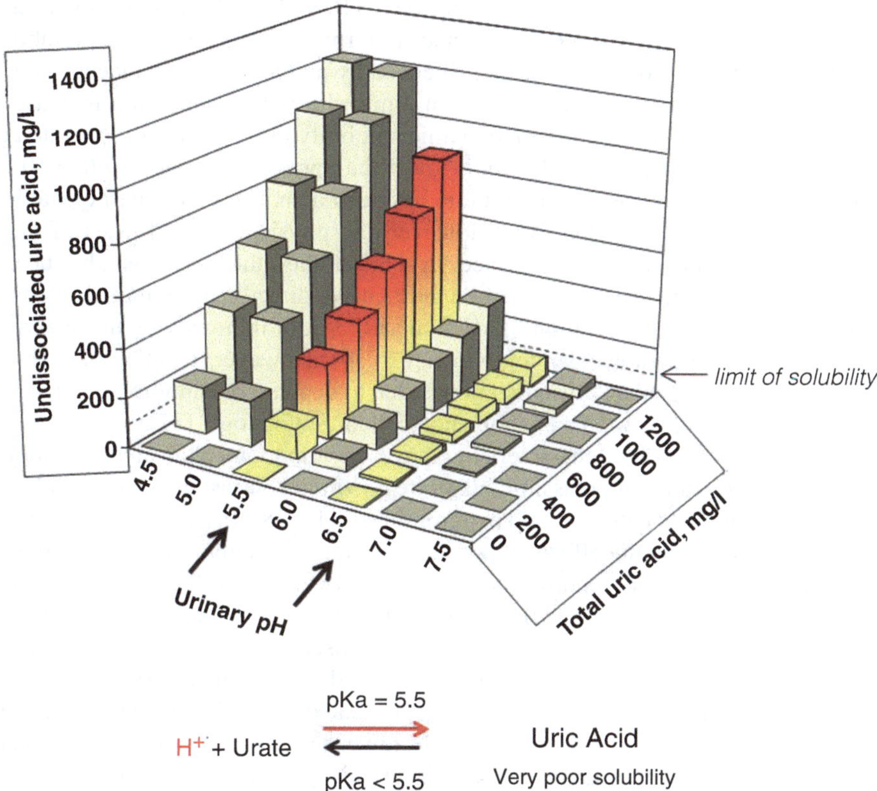



**Fig. 7.3** Significance of urinary pH in uric acid solubility

pH of $5.40 \pm 0.23$ compared with normal subjects at $5.96 \pm 0.47$ and low fractional urinary uric acid excretion. In another inpatient study consisting of ten subjects with pure uric acid stones, urinary uric acid of $540 \pm 322$ was not different from the urinary uric acid of normal subjects at $657 \pm 337$ [30]. Similarly, in 56 patients with idiopathic uric acid nephrolithiasis who underwent a full outpatient evaluation with an ad lib diet, uric acid stone formers had significantly lower urinary uric acid, significantly lower fractional excretion of uric acid, and significantly higher serum uric acid levels compared with a control group comprising 54 patients with hypercalciuria and two normal subjects, matched for age, BMI, and gender [31]. These studies support the principle that an important determinant for the formation of uric acid stones is unduly acidic urine.

Limited solubility of 96 mg/L at urinary pH ranging between 4.4 and 5.5 requires a total uric acid concentration (undissociated + urate) of 110–200 mg/L to exceed its solubility limits. However, at a urinary pH of 6.2–6.4 the total uric acid concentration should exceed 1,100 mg/L in order to precipitate (Fig. 7.3). Furthermore, under normal physiologic circumstances it is not anticipated that urinary uric acid excretion demonstrates such wide variations between 110 and 1,100 mg/day. However, urinary pH between 4.6 and 6.6 is expected in normal subjects. Uric acid solubility in the urinary environment is also influenced by ambient cation concentrations [32]. It has been demonstrated that sodium diminishes while potassium increases urate solubility [19, 32]. The thermodynamic solubility product of sodium urate at $2.79 \times 10^{-5}$ M$^2$ was found to be 3.5-folds lower than potassium urate at $9.63 \times 10^{-5}$ M$^2$ [32, 33]. Moreover, monosodium urate has been demonstrated to participate in calcium oxalate crystallization [34]. However, the physicochemical basis of this process has not yet been well established. In some studies, the mechanism has been attributed to calcium salt crystallization influenced directly by epitaxial crystal growth, heterogeneous nucleation of calcium salt [34], or indirectly by the adsorption of urinary macromolecular inhibitors [35, 36]. However, another study has shown that calcium oxalate crystallization is due to decreased solubility of calcium oxalate in a solution, through a phenomenon called "salting out" [37].

These physicochemical characteristics have an important clinical implication showing the superiority of potassium-alkali treatment in contrast with sodium-alkali treatment in patients with uric acid nephrolithiasis [19, 38]. In a metabolically balanced study comparing the effects of potassium citrate and sodium-citrate therapies in patients with uric acid nephrolithiasis, it was shown that both alkali treatments significantly increased urinary pH. However, the potassium-alkali treatment lowered urinary calcium significantly and markedly raised urinary citrate. As a result, the urinary saturation of calcium oxalate diminished significantly during this treatment and the inhibitor activity against calcium oxalate significantly increased. In contrast, sodium citrate did not significantly lower urinary calcium and increased saturation of monosodium urate. The rise in urinary pH with sodium-alkali therapy was similar to potassium-alkali treatment (Table 7.1). As a result of the above changes, both alkali therapies were equally effective in preventing the propensity for uric acid stone formation since their ability to increase urinary pH was similar. However, potassium-alkali treatment has advantages over sodium-alkali therapy by lowering urinary calcium and raising urinary citrate without raising urinary supersaturation with respect to monosodium urate, thereby preventing the risk of calcium oxalate precipitation [19] (see Table 7.1).


## Treatment Approach

### *Alkali Treatment*

#### Idiopathic Uric Acid Nephrolithiasis

Uric acid nephrolithiasis is principally the disease of urinary pH. Despite the lack of a large randomized, placebo-controlled study, one open-ended trial in 18 patients with uric acid nephrolithiasis, comprising six patients with isolated uric acid stones and 12 with mixed uric acid and/or calcium oxalate stones who

**Table 7.1** Comparison of biochemical and physiochemical profiles of potassium citrate and sodium citrate

|  | Potassium citrate | Sodium citrate |
|---|---|---|
| Urine pH | ↑ | ↑ |
| Urine citrate | ↑ | ↑ |
| Urine calcium | ↓ | ↑ |
| Urine sodium | ↔ | ↑ |
| Urine potassium | ↑ | ↔ |
| Supersaturation profiles |  |  |
| Potassium urate | ↑ | = |
| Sodium urate | ↔ | ↑ |
| Calcium oxalate | ↓↓ | ↓ |
| Inhibitor activity against calcium oxalate crystallization | ↑ | ↔ |
| Prevention of uric acid stones | ↓ | ↓ |
| Prevention of calcium oxalate stones | ↓↓ | ↔ |

↑ = increased, ↓ = decreased, ↓↓ = prominent decrease, ↔ = normal/ no change

received long-term treatment (mean of 2.7–8 years) with potassium-alkali treatment (average of 60 mEq/day), demonstrated a significant rise in urinary pH and a significant fall in urinary content of undissociated uric acid to the normal range [38] (Fig. 7.4). Potassium-citrate treatment was associated with a significant rise in urinary citrate and a fall in urinary saturation of calcium oxalate. Moreover, the new stone-formation rate declined significantly from $1.20 \pm 1.68$ stones/year to $0.01 \pm 0.04$ stones/year during treatment (Fig. 7.5). In five patients with pure uric acid stones, stone formation recurred following treatment with sodium alkali. Stone analysis revealed the transformation from uric acid to calcium oxalate and calcium phosphate stones. However, treatment with potassium alkali over 1–3.5 years resulted in no new stone events. The result of this study provided sufficient evidence of the therapeutic efficacy of potassium-citrate treatment in the management of uric acid nephrolithiasis. The improvement in urinary biochemical crystallization profiles was associated with the significant remission in stone events.

In clinical practice, the average dosage of alkali used in the treatment of uric acid nephrolithiasis ranges between 30 and 60 mEq/day. This is based on the principle that optimal intake of protein in the population is 0.8 g/kg body weight per day. Approximately 1 mEq of hydrogen is produced by 1 g of protein; therefore, in average individuals with 70 kg body weight, approximately 60 mEq of alkali is sufficient to neutralize the acid load produced by protein. In a previous study in 18 patients with uric acid nephrolithiasis, when urinary pH increased from 5.30 to normal (6.19–6.46) during alkali treatment, urinary content of undissociated uric acid decreased to normal range (64–108 mg/day) [38]. Given that urinary uric acid in both ad lib and fixed metabolic diets does not exceed 545–657 mg/day [15, 31], treatment with alkali alone is sufficient to lower the risk of uric acid precipitation and kidney stone formation. In rare exceptions, when urinary uric acid excretion exceeds 1,000–2,000 mg, in such a prevailing urinary pH environment, treatment with a hypouricosuric agent maybe necessary [39].

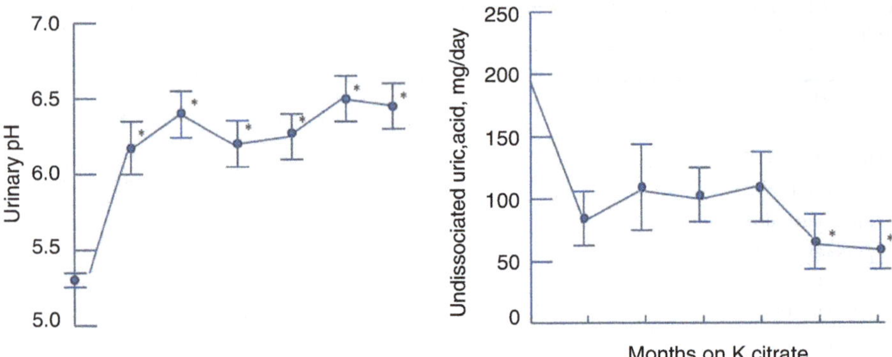


**Fig. 7.4** Effect of potassium-citrate treatment on urinary pH and undissociated uric acid in patients with uric acid nephrolithiasis. Significant difference from pretreatment value produced by treatment is shown by * for $p < 0.05$. (Reprinted with permission from Macmillan Publishers Ltd. [38])

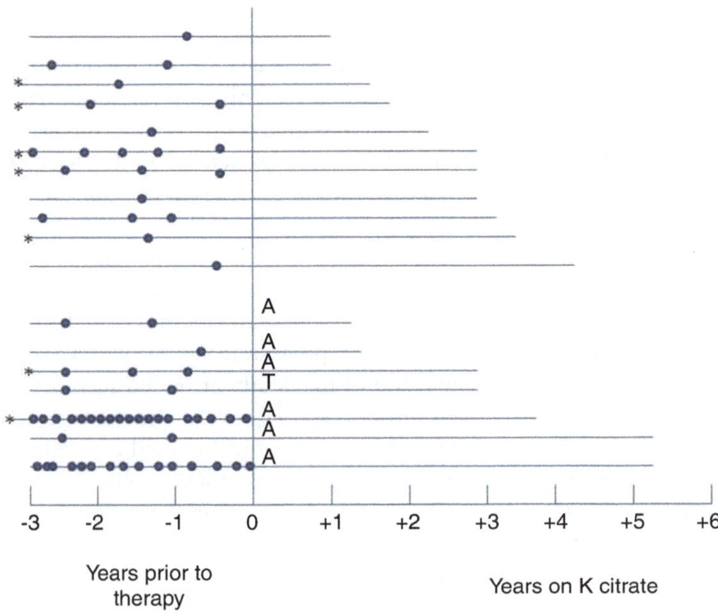


**Fig. 7.5** Effect of potassium-citrate treatment on new stone formation in patients with uric acid nephrolithiasis. Each *circle* represents new stone formation. Each *line* indicates study in a separate patient. *Asterisk* denotes patients with preexisting stone when the treatment with potassium citrate was begun. Bottom seven patients took potassium citrate concurrently with allopurinol (*A*) or thiazide (*T*). (Reprinted with permission from Macmillan Publishers Ltd. [38])

The diurnal variation in urinary acidification differs among normal individuals and uric acid stone formers. A recent metabolic study [30] has shown that throughout the day, both normal and uric acid stone formers show significant variation in urinary pH. Urinary pH increases in the morning, peaks at noon, falls after lunch, and rises again during the afternoon only to fall again after the evening meal. During the night, urine pH decreases until 6 a.m. before rising again in the morning. However, throughout the day urine pH remains significantly lower in uric acid stone formers compared to normal subjects [30]. Thus, it seems logical to suggest that one dose of alkali treatment must be given at bedtime to overcome undue urine acidity during nighttime and reduce the risk of uric acid precipitation [40]. Occasionally, carbonic anhydrase inhibitors (Diamox) have been used as an alternative alkalinizing agent [41]. However, such a treatment must be used cautiously due to the development of systemic acidosis, hypocitraturia, and highly alkaline urine, which is a risk for the increase of calcium phosphate stone formation [42, 43].

**Chronic Diarrheal States**

In inflammatory bowel diseases including ulcerative colitis and Crohn's disease, the majority of stones contain calcium. However, one-thirds of stones are composed of uric acid, an incidence that is higher than reported at 8.5 - 10% in general populations with uric acid nephrolithiasis [24, 44, 45]. Moreover, in patients following ileostomy, uric acid stones are common and comprise two-thirds of all stones [24]. In these subjects, unduly acidic urine pH (<5.5) is commonly encountered compared to control subjects [46–48]. However, urinary uric acid excretion has been reported to be normal in this population [49]. The underlying pathophysiologic mechanism for undue urine acidity in this population has not yet been fully investigated. The major therapeutic modality in these subjects should involve administration of alkali treatment to combat abnormally acidic urine [49] in conjunction with increased intake of fluids, as urine volume is significantly low due to persistent diarrheal fluid loss.

## Treatment with Hypouricosuric Agents

Treatment with uric acid-lowering drugs (allopurinol) is commonly required in hyperuricosuric conditions as stated below. One alternative agent is Febuxostat, which is a new xanthine oxidase inhibitor.

**Primary Gout**

The incidence of uric acid stones in patients with primary gout is directly proportionate to the amount of urinary uric acid excretion [50]. In addition to hyperuricosuria, urinary pH has been reported to be low in this population [20]. The genetic basis of primary gout has not yet been identified. However, it has been demonstrated that primary gout has familial incidence of approximately 30 % [20, 50].

## Genetic Disturbances in Uric Acid Metabolic Pathways

Characteristically, subjects with monogenic enzymatic disorders in purine metabolism show a significantly elevated rate of uric acid production and, consequently, elevated serum uric acid and urinary uric acid exceeding 10 mg/dL and 1,000 mg/day, respectively. More than two-thirds of this population suffer from uric acid stones, usually before the third decade of life. The three well-defined enzymatic disorders in uric acid metabolism pathways are (1) hypoxanthine guanine phosphoribosyltranferase deficiency (Lesch–Nyhan syndrome), (2) phosphoribosylpyrophosphate synthase overactivity, and (3) glucose-six-phosphatase deficiency [51]. Some of the clinical manifestations in Lesch–Nyhan syndrome, such as neurologic complications, may appear in the first years of life. However, crystalluria and hematuria may be present in the first months of life, thereby leading to kidney injury [52]. In another monogenic enzymatic disorder, patients may suffer from adenine phosphoribosyltranferase deficiency. In such an enzymatic effect, adenine is converted to 8-hydroxyadenine, which is further metabolized to dihydroxyadenine, which leads to dihydroxyadenine stone formation and nephropathy [53]. These stones, much like uric acid stones, are radiolucent in nature but are biochemically distinct. Unlike in Lesch–Nyhan syndrome cases, in those with adenine phosphoribosyltranferase deficiency, complications may occur at any age, which presents challenges for diagnosis. The diagnosis is made by identification of crystals in the urine or by stone analysis. Stones should be analyzed by morphologic assessment under a stereomicroscope and with infrared spectroscopy, since biochemical stone analysis does not differentiate these types of stones from uric acid stones.

The principle treatment for this disorder is allopurinol, which has been shown to improve and stabilize renal function, unlike treatment in patients with hypoxanthine guanine phosphoribosyltranferase deficiency. In these monogenic enzymatic disorders, alkalinization of the urine is not recommended, since impaired urinary acidification has not been detected and treatment with alkali is not necessary in some instances, like dihydroxyadenine stones due to the lack of solubility and urinary pH > 8.5.

## Increased Tissue Turnover

In numerous disease states, such as myeloproliferative disorders and hemolytic anemia, hyperuricosuria in excess of 1,000 mg/day and serum uric acid levels > 10 mg/dL occur due to increased tissue breakdown [54]. In this population, secondary gout is commonly associated with recurrent uric acid stones and uric acid nephropathy, consequently causing significant morbidity and mortality. The result of allopurinol treatment in 16 out of 63 patients was rewarding, as this treatment virtually stopped kidney stone formation [54].

**Acknowledgments** The author would like to acknowledge Ashlei L. Johnson for her primary role in the preparation and editorial review of this manuscript.

The author was supported by the National Institutes of Health Grant R01-DK81423.

# References


1. Mandel NS, Mandel GS. Urinary tract stone disease in the United States veteran population. 2. Geographical analysis of variations in composition. J Urol. 1989;142:1516–21.
2. Pak CY, Sakhaee K, Moe O, Preminger GM, Poindexter JR, Peterson RD, et al. Biochemical profile of stone-forming patients with diabetes mellitus. Urology. 2003;61:523–7.
3. Lieske JC, de la Vega LS, Gettman MT, Slezak JM, Bergstralh EJ, Melton LJ 3rd, et al. Diabetes mellitus and the risk of urinary tract stones: a population-based case-control study. AM J Kidney Dis. 2006;48:897–904.
4. Ekeruo WO, Tan YH, Young MD, Dahm P, Maloney ME, Mathias BJ, et al. Metabolic risk factors and the impact of medical therapy on the management of nephrolithiasis in obese patients. J Urol. 2004;172:159–63.
5. Daudon M, Lacour B, Jungers P. Influence of body size on urinary stone composition in men and women. Urol Res. 2006;34:193–9.
6. Daudon M, Traxer O, Conort P, Lacour B, Jungers P. Type 2 diabetes increases the risk for uric acid stones. J Am Soc Nephrol. 2006;17:2026–33.
7. Portis AJ, Hermans K, Culhane-Pera KA, Curhan GC. Stone disease in the Hmong of Minnesota: initial description of a high-risk population. J Endourol. 2004;18:853–7.
8. Portis AJ, Laliberte M, Tatman P, Moua M, Culhane-Pera K, Maalouf NM, et al. High prevalence of gouty arthritis among the Hmong population in Minnesota. Arthritis Care Res (Hoboken). 2010;62:1386–91.
9. Cameron MA, Maalouf NM, Adams-Huet B, Moe OW, Sakhaee K. Urine composition in type 2 diabetes: predisposition to uric acid nephrolithiasis. J Am Soc Nephrol. 2006;17:1422–8.
10. Prasongwatana V, Sriboonlue P, Suntarapa S. Urinary stone composition in North-East Thailand. Br J Urol. 1983;55:353–5.
11. Herbstein FH, Kleeberg J, Shalitin Y, Wartski E, Wielinski S. Chemical and x-ray diffraction analysis of urinary stones in Israel. Isr J Med Sci. 1974;10:1493–9.
12. Sakhaee K. Uric acid metabolism and uric acid stones. In: Rao NP, Preminger GM, Kavanagh JP, editors. Urinary tract stone disease. Manchester: Springer; 2011.p. 185–93.
13. Sakhaee K. Recent advances in the pathophysiology of nephrolithiasis. Kidney Int. 2009;75:585–95.
14. Rafey MA, Lipkowitz MS, Leal-Pinto E, Abramson RG. Uric acid transport. Curr Opin Nephrol Hypertens. 2003;12:511–6.
15. Sakhaee K, Adams-Huet B, Moe OW, Pak CY. Pathophysiologic basis for normouricosuric uric acid nephrolithiasis. Kidney Int. 2002;62:971–9.
16. Asplin JR. Uric acid stones. Sem Nep. 1996;16:412–24.
17. Coe FL, Strauss AL, Tembe V, Le Dun S. Uric acid saturation in calcium nephrolithiasis. Kidney Int. 1980;17:662–8.
18. Finlayson B, Smith A. Stability of first dissociable proton of uric acid. J Chem Eng Data. 1974;19:94–7.
19. Sakhaee K, Nicar M, Hill K, Pak CY. Contrasting effects of potassium citrate and sodium citrate therapies on urinary chemistries and crystallization of stone-forming salts. Kidney Int. 1983;24:348–52.
20. Gutman AB, Yu TF. Uric acid nephrolithiasis. Am J Med. 1968;45:756–79.
21. Pak CY, Moe OW, Sakhaee K, Peterson RD, Poindexter JR. Physicochemical metabolic characteristics for calcium oxalate stone formation in patients with gouty diathesis. J Urol. 2005;173:1606–9.
22. Kok DJ, Papapoulos SE, Bijvoet OL. Excessive crystal agglomeration with low citrate excretion in recurrent stone-formers. Lancet. 1986;1:1056–8.
23. Sakhaee K, Nigam S, Snell P, Hsu MC, Pak CY. Assessment of the pathogenetic role of physical exercise in renal stone formation. J Clin Endocrinol Metab. 1987;65:974–79.
24. Deren JJ, Porush JG, Levitt MF, Khilnani MT. Nephrolithiasis as a complication of ulcerative colitis and regional enteritis. Ann Intern Med. 1962;56:843–53.

25. Moe OW, Abate N, Sakhaee K. Pathophysiology of uric acid nephrolithiasis. Endocrinol Metab Clin North Am. 2002;31:895–914.
26. Tanaka M, Itoh K, Matsushita K, Matsushita K, Wakita N, Adachi M, et al. Two male siblings with hereditary renal hypouricemia and exercise-induced ARF. Am J Kidney Dis. 2003;42:1287–92.
27. Ichida K, Hosoyamada M, Hisatome I, Enomoto A, Hikita M, Endou H, et al. Clinical and molecular analysis of patients with renal hypouricemia in Japan-influence of URAT1 gene on urinary urate excretion. J Am Soc Nephrol. 2004;15:164–73.
28. Maalouf NM, Sakhaee K, Parks JH, Coe FL, Adams-Huet B, Pak CY. Association of urinary pH with body weight in nephrolithiasis. Kidney Int. 2004;65:1422–5.
29. Maalouf NM, Cameron MA, Moe OW, Sakhaee K. Metabolic basis for low urine pH in type 2 diabetes. Clin J Am Soc Nephrol. 2010;5:1277–81.
30. Cameron M, Maalouf NM, Poindexter J, Adams-Huet B, Sakhaee K, Moe OW. The diurnal variation in urine acidification differs between normal individuals and uric acid stone formers. Kidney Int. 2012;81:1123–30.
31. Pak CY, Sakhaee K, Peterson RD, Poindexter JR, Frawley WH. Biochemical profile of idiopathic uric acid nephrolithiasis. Kidney Int. 2001;60:757–61.
32. Pak CY, Waters O, Arnold L, Holt K, Cox C, Barilla D. Mechanism for calcium urolithiasis among patients with hyperuricosuria: supersaturation of urine with respect to monosodium urate. J Clin Invest. 1977;59:426–31.
33. Pak C, Holt K, Britton F, Peterson R, Crother C, Ward D. Assesment of pathogenetic role of uric acid, monpotassium urate, monoammonium urate, monosodium urate in hyperuricosuric calcium oxalate nephrolithiasis Miner Electrolyte Metab. 1980;4:130–6.
34. Pak CY, Arnold LH. Heterogeneous nucleation of calcium oxalate by seeds of monosodium urate. Proc Soc Exp Biol Med. 1975;149:930–2.
35. Lonsdale K. Epitaxy as a growth factor in urinary calculi and gallstones. Nature. 1968;217:56–8.
36. Zerwekh JE, Holt K, Pak CY. Natural urinary macromolecular inhibitors: attenuation of inhibitory activity by urate salts. Kidney Int. 1983;23:838–41.
37. Grover PK, Ryall RL. Urate and calcium oxalate stones: from repute to rhetoric to reality. Miner Electrolyte Metab. 1994;20:361–70.
38. Pak CY, Sakhaee K, Fuller C. Successful management of uric acid nephrolithiasis with potassium citrate. Kidney Int. 1986;30:422–8.
39. Maalouf NM, Cameron MA, Moe OW, Sakhaee K. Novel insights into the pathogenesis of uric acid nephrolithiasis. Curr Opin Nephrol Hypertens. 2004;13:181–9.
40. Cameron MA, Baker LA, Maalouf NM, Moe OW, Sakhaee K. Circadian variation in urine pH and uric acid nephrolithiasis risk. Nephrol Dial Transplant. 2007;22:2375–8.
41. Freed SZ. The alternating use of an alkalizing salt and acetazolamide in the management of cystine and uric acid stones. J Urol. 1975;113:96–9.
42. Gordon EE, Sheps SG. Effect of acetazolamide on citrate excretion and formation of renal calculi. N Engl J Med. 1957;256:1215–9.
43. Kuo RL, Moran ME, Kim DH, Abrahams HM, White MD, Lingeman JE. Topiramate-induced nephrolithiasis. J Endourol. 2002;16:229–31.
44. Gelzayd EA, Breuer RI, Kirsner JB. Nephrolithiasis in inflammatory bowel disease. Am J Dig Dis. 1968;13:1027–34.
45. Knudsen L, Marcussen H, Fleckenstein P, Pedersen EB, Jarnum S. Urolithiasis in chronic inflammatory bowel disease. Scand J Gastroenterol. 1978;13:433–6.
46. Bambach CP, Robertson WG, Peacock M, Hill GL. Effect of intestinal surgery on the risk of urinary stone formation. Gut. 1981;22:257–63.
47. Fukushima T, Yamazaki Y, Sugita A, Tsuchiya S. Prophylaxis of uric acid stone in patients with inflammatory bowel disease following extensive colonic resection. Gastroenterol Jpn. 1991;26:430–4.
48. Clarke AM, McKenzie RG. Ileostomy and the risk of urinary uric acid stones. Lancet. 1969;2:395–7.

49. Obialo CI, Clayman RV, Matts JP, Fitch LL, Buchwald H, Gillis M, et al. Pathogenesis of nephrolithiasis post-partial ileal bypass surgery: case-control study. The POSCH Group. Kidney Int. 1991;39:1249–54.
50. Yu T, Gutman AB. Uric acid nephrolithiasis in gout. Predisposing factors. Ann Intern Med. 1967;67:1133–48.
51. Wyngaarden JB, Kelley WN. Gout. In: Stanbury JB, Wyngaarden JB, Frederickson DS, editors. The metabolic basis of inherited disease. 3rd ed. New York: McGraw-Hill; 1972.p. 889–968.
52. Roche A, Perez-Duenas B, Camacho JA, Torres RJ, Puig JG, García-Cazorla A, et al. Efficacy of rasburicase in hyperuricemia secondary to Lesch-Nyhan syndrome. Am J Kidney Dis. 2009;53:677–80.
53. Bollee G, Harambat J, Bensman A, Knebelmann B, Daudon M, Ceballos-Picot I. Adenine phosphoribosyltransferase deficiency. Clin J Am Soc Nephrol. 2012;7:1521–7.
54. Yu T, Weinreb N, Wittman R, Wasserman LR. Secondary gout associated with chronic myeloproliferative disorders. Semin Arthritis Rheum. 1976;5:247–56.

# Chapter 8
# Cystinuria: Assessing and Managing Risk

Nicola T. Sumorok and David S. Goldfarb

## Introduction

Cystinuria is a rare, inherited form of nephrolithiasis. It is caused by impaired reabsorption of cystine, a homodimer of the amino acid cysteine, by renal proximal tubular cells. Due to its insolubility, the decreased reabsorption of filtered cystine leads to cystine nephrolithiasis. Impaired reabsorption of ornithine, lysine, and arginine also occurs, but the increased excretion of these dibasic amino acids has no clinical consequence. This disorder is the result of the inheritance of genetic mutations in genes that code for the proteins which form an amino acid transporter located in the apical membrane of the proximal tubular epithelial cells of the kidney and in the small intestine. The two genes that are responsible for the defective transporter in patients with cystinuria are *SLC3A1* and *SCL7A9*.

Although cystinuria is an inherited disease, there are clearly many factors that contribute to stone formation, as there is a wide variation in stone occurrence both from patient to patient, and across a patient's lifetime. We are aware of some of the risk factors that contribute to stone formation in these patients, such as dietary factors and the amount of fluid intake, that affect the urinary chemistry and cystine concentration in the urine, respectively. There may also be factors that we are unaware of that contribute to the risk. Current methods of assessing a patient's risk include analyses of the urine, such as urine volume, urinary pH, and measurements of urinary cystine, sodium, and urea nitrogen. A thorough history including dietary and fluid intake history, medications, and information regarding environmental factors,

D. S. Goldfarb (✉)
Nephrology, New York Harbor VA Healthcare System, NYU Langone Medical Center,
423 E. 23rd St./111G, New York, NY 10010,USA
e-mail: david.goldfarb@va.gov

N. T. Sumorok
Medical Service, New York Harbor VA Healthcare System, NYU Langone Medical Center,
423 E. 23rd St., New York, NY 10010, USA
e-mail: nicols01@nyumc.org

M. S. Pearle, S. Y. Nakada (eds.), *Practical Controversies in Medical Management
of Stone Disease,* DOI 10.1007/978-1-4614-9575-8_8,
© Springer Science+Business Media New York 2014

such as occupational conditions, is also important in assessing the patient's overall risk of stone formation and determining areas of potential intervention.


## Genetics and Epidemiology

In 1994, linkage analyses identified *SLC3A1* on the short arm of chromosome 2 as the first defective gene known to cause cystinuria. *SLC3A1* codes for a 663-amino acid heavy subunit of the cystine transporter, rBAT ("related to $b^{0,+}$ amino acid transporter"). A second gene mutation, *SCL7A9*, located on the long arm of chromosome 19, was found in 1999. *SCL7A9* codes for a 487-amino acid light subunit of the cystine transporter called $b^{0,+}$ AT (amino acid transporter of neutral and positively charged particles). Together, the two subunits are linked by a disulfide bridge to form a heterodimer which is located in the apical membrane of the proximal tubule cells. To date, 135 mutations in *SCL3A1* and 95 mutations in *SCL7A9* have been identified [1]. rBAT is the "helper" protein which traffics $b^{0,+}$ AT, the catalytic transport protein, to the apical membrane of the proximal tubule.

Although cystinuria accounts for no more than 1 % of all renal calculi, it is one of the most common inherited genetic diseases. It is estimated that the gene occurs in about 0.01 % of people, with an average worldwide prevalence of about 1 in 7,000 people. There is a significant variation in prevalence by population, with a prevalence as high as 1 in 2,500 people among Libyan Jews, and as low as 1 in 100,000 people in Sweden [2]. In the USA, the prevalence is estimated to be approximately 1 in 15,000; however, these figures likely underestimate the true prevalence because some patients with cystinuria do not form stones, and therefore escape detection. Additionally, due to its low prevalence among stone formers, the diagnosis may be overlooked if stone analysis is not completed.


## Classification

Traditionally, patients with cystinuria were classified on the basis of the urinary cystine excretion pattern of their parents, or obligate heterozygotes. Heterozygotes of type I cystinuria had normal urinary cystine excretion patterns (0–100 μmoles of cystine per gram of creatinine), whereas heterozygotes of type II and type III (later called non-type I) were characterized by an increase in urinary cystine excretion [3]. Once the genes for cystinuria were identified, it was thought that mutations in *SLC3A1* were responsible for type I as a result of the defective rBAT protein, and that non-type I cystinuria was due to mutations in *SLC7A9*, and the resulting defective $b^{0,+}$ AT subunit of the amino-acid transporter. The less severe phenotype in heterozygotes with *SLC3A1* disease was explained by the difference in function between the two subunits of the transporter [1]. A study by Della Strologo showed that urinary excretion patterns of heterozygotes did not accurately predict the type of mutation in 14% of cases, so the traditional phenotypic classification system has been replaced by a genotypic one [3]. Patients with two SLC3A1 mutations are classified as having type A cystinuria, whereas patients with two SLC7A9 mutations have type B cystinuria. Only a very small subset of patients (1.6% of the study population) was found to have one mutation in each gene, or type AB disease. Cystinuria has usually been considered an autosomal recessive disease. However, because patients heterozygous for SLC7A9 mutations have increased amounts of cystine excretion, not usually but perhaps sometimes sufficient to cause stones, cystinuria may also be considered an example of an "incomplete dominant" disease. Patients with the rare type AB cystinuria have two mutated alleles in one gene and one mutated allele in the other, so they are actually type AAB or ABB. One mutation in each allele (AB) does not result in phenotypic disease, thereby ruling out digenic inheritance [4].

This somewhat complex mode of genetic inheritance makes estimating the risk of a patient with cystinuria passing on the disorder to his/her offspring difficult to determine without knowing the underlying genetic mutations. We rarely perform genetic testing for cystinuria though it is likely that less expensive testing will soon be widely available. In general we advise young people with cystinuria that their likelihood of reproducing with a carrier of a mutated gene is about 1/170. Half of their children would then be expected to have two mutated genes and have the stone-forming phenotype while the other 50% would be carriers. Whether the carriers would have abnormal cystine excretion would depend on whether the mutated gene was *SCL3A1* in which case they would have no cystine in the urine, or *SLC7A9* in which case they would.

## Diagnosis and Testing

There are several different methods of diagnosing patients with cystinuria. Examination of the urinalysis will lead to the diagnosis in approximately 25% of patients with cystinuria, by the identification of the pathognomonic hexagonal-shaped cystine crystals. Historically, a cyanide-nitroprusside test was used as a screening tool. Although it is not 100% specific, it detects cystine in the urine by displaying a red–purple color change when the reduced sulfhydryl groups that form from mixing cystine and cyanide react with nitroprusside. A definitive diagnosis of cystinuria is made by analysis of stone composition. In patients in whom this is not available, an alternative method is quantification of urinary cystine on a 24-h urine sample. Normal urinary cystine excretion is typically less than 30 mg per day, whereas patients with cystinuria will excrete >250 mg per day. SLC7A9 heterozygotes will show an increase in urinary cystine excretion, usually in between 30 and 250 mg per day. Genetic testing can also confirm the diagnosis; however, as stated above, it is not routinely performed if the diagnosis is made by other means because it is unlikely to affect clinical management.

Once a diagnosis of cystinuria is made, patients are followed by both imaging studies that assess stone burden, and urine tests that monitor cystine excretion.

Although the direct measurement of urinary cystine has been used clinically to date, it is inaccurate for several reasons. Patients with acid urine pH will precipitate cystine which will escape measurement; urine collections should be routinely alkalinized by the lab before cystine is assayed [5]. In addition, many cystine assays measure free sulfhydryl groups using colorimetric reactions. These reactions do not reliably distinguish cystine from soluble thiol-cysteine drug complexes, so they cannot accurately measure cystine in the presence of cystine-binding thiol drugs (CBTDs) such as D-penicillamine and tiopronin. Other techniques, such as high-performance liquid chromatography (HPLC) can distinguish between the two, but the preparation of the sample for HPLC may lead to disruption of the thiol drug-cysteine complex [6]. This again leads to inaccurate measurements of cystine in the presence of CBTDs. Even in the absence of CBTDs, measurement of cystine supersaturation cannot reliably be calculated from the measurement of cystine concentration and urine pH [5]. Nakagawa et al. demonstrated in their in vitro study that there was a large variability of cystine solubility at different pH values.

These problems led to the development of a new assay called cystine capacity that directly measures the ability of a patient's urine to solubilize or precipitate cystine [7]. It is a "solid phase assay" in which a prefixed amount of cystine crystals are added to a patient's urine. After incubation for 48 h, the urine is spun and the supernatant removed so that the amount of solid cystine can be measured. In supersaturated urine, cystine precipitates onto the added crystals, so the solid phase that is recovered is greater than that which was added. The amount of cystine added to the crystals is quantified and reported as a negative number, or a "negative cystine capacity." Undersaturated urine can dissolve the added cystine crystals; such urine has a "positive cystine capacity." This test is now commercially available in the USA, performed by Litholink (Chicago, IL). A clinical trial is underway to evaluate its ability to accurately predict the development of kidney stones. In this prospective study, patients with cystinuria undergo biannual imaging studies to monitor stone formation and perform 24-h urine collections every 6 months for cystine capacity measurements. The hope is that the assay can accurately predict risk of stone formation so that physicians can use it to adjust preventive therapy.

## Long-term Risks

Several population-based cohort studies have shown that patients with symptomatic kidney stones are at increased risk of developing chronic kidney disease compared to the general population [8]. The mechanism of injury is thought to be secondary to obstructive uropathy or pyelonephritis; however, crystal plugs at the ducts of Bellini and parenchymal injury from shockwave lithotripsy may also contribute. Among stone formers, cystinuric patients have been shown to have lower creatinine clearances compared to patients with other types of nephrolithiasis [9]. A possible explanation for this is the early-age onset of stone formation in cystinuria and the need for multiple urologic procedures. A study by Assimos et al. supports this theory. In this retrospective cohort study, calcium oxalate stone formers were compared to people with cystinuria. Mean serum creatinine was found to be significantly higher in stone-forming cystinurics compared to calcium oxalate stone formers, and male gender, increasing number of open surgical stone removing procedures and nephrectomy were significant variables associated with an increased serum creatinine [10]. However, patients with Dent disease, primary hyperoxaluria and dihydroxyadenine stones had worse reductions in kidney function [11].

## Treatment

The overall goal of treatment of cystinuria is prevention of recurrent kidney stone formation, both to decrease morbidity and to minimize the risk of developing chronic kidney disease in the long term. This is achieved through several mechanisms, including increasing the solubility of cystine by increasing urine pH, decreasing the concentration of cystine by limiting consumption of its precursors and increasing fluid intake, and converting cystine to the more soluble form monomer cysteine. In practice, we typically start with fluid therapy and dietary modifications. Alkalinizing agents are added in order to increase the urine pH to its target in most patients. Finally, medications such as CBTDs are reserved for patients who are refractory to the above interventions. Although these medications, in our experience, are better tolerated than one might have been led to believe, they do have side effects that lead to their less frequent prescription than alkali.

As in all etiologies of nephrolithiasis, fluid therapy to decrease urinary concentration of cystine remains one of the mainstays of therapy. The goal is to decrease urinary cystine concentration to less than 250 mg/L, if possible. Patients with cystinuria often excrete greater than 1 g of cystine per day, which therefore requires greater than 4 L fluid intake per day to achieve that goal. To be effective, it is important to maintain high urine flow rates over all 24 h of the day. Therefore, drinking fluid at bedtime should be encouraged, even if sleep is (slightly) interrupted by nocturia, to prevent nocturnal aggregation of crystals. Environmental and occupational factors may play a role in how effective or successful fluid therapy can be. Patients who live in warmer climates or spend a significant amount of time outside in the sun may require even more fluid intake to maintain a high urine output due to insensible losses from the heat. Occupations can limit a patient's ability to increase their fluid intake. For example, teachers may not be able to leave a classroom to urinate frequently throughout the day, and therefore are limited in the amount of fluid they can drink. In these circumstances, medications become more important in preventing stone formation.

Alkalinization of the urine, increasing its pH, is another therapeutic goal in the prevention of stone formation in patients with cystinuria. As shown by Dent et al. over 50 years ago, the solubility of cystine increases significantly with increases in urine pH. In these early studies, cystine was found to have a solubility of < 300 mg/L at a urine pH of 7.0, which was increased to 500 mg/L at a pH of 7.5 [12]. This find-

**Fig. 8.1** Cystine solubility (mmol/L) was strongly
correlated with urine pH.
*Circles*: men; *triangles*:
women; *open symbols*: no
thiol drugs; *closed symbols*:
with thiols. *Ellipses* enclose
1 standard deviation from the
mean; *solid line*: men; *broken
line*: women. (Reproduced
with permission from [13])

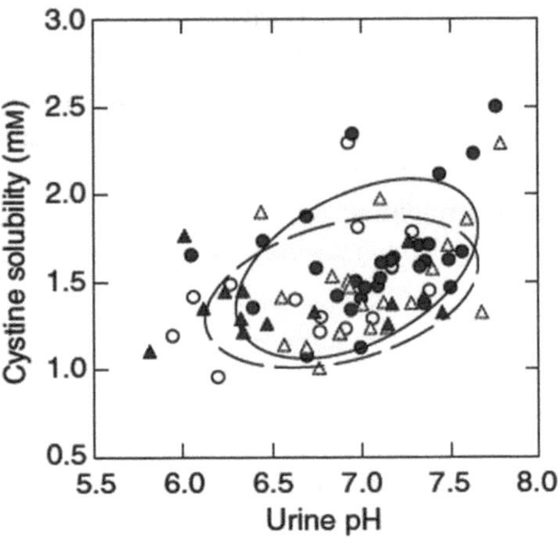


ing has been replicated in subsequent studies. In 91 urine samples from 64 patients
with cystinuria, it was clearly demonstrated that alkalinization of urine increases
the solubility of cystine [13] (Fig. 8.1). Alkalinization is usually achieved with
medications such as potassium citrate or sodium citrate, but can also be affected by
lowering dietary intake of animal protein, which represents an acid load. The goal
urine pH is usually greater than 7.5, although this may be limited by the increased
risk of forming calcium phosphate stones that comes with a higher urine pH. This
occurs very infrequently as citrate itself inhibits calcium phosphate crystallization
and diminishes urine calcium excretion, while the prescribed large urine volumes
further reduce risk. Litholink provides a summary of stone risk through analysis of
24-h urine samples that includes the supersaturation of calcium phosphate in addition to urinary cystine levels and cystine capacity, so that practitioners can monitor
this risk while prescribing alkali therapy.

Dietary protein restriction not only decreases the acid load, but also decreases
the amount of methionine consumed, which is the amino acid precursor for cystine.
A study of seven cystinuric patients on a metabolic ward compared the urinary cystine excretion on a high-protein diet to a low-protein diet. The results showed that
a low-protein diet decreased the mean excretion of cystine from 6.1 to 4.9 mmol
in 24 h compared to a high-protein diet [14]. A recent study also showed that the
amount of urinary urea nitrogen excretion, a surrogate for protein intake, significantly correlates with urinary cystine excretion [13] (Fig. 8.2). As a result of these
findings, patients with cystinuria on diets that are high in animal protein may benefit from a more vegetarian diet.

Salt restriction is another dietary modification that is important in preventing
stone formation in patients with cystinuria. Although the reabsorption of cystine
is independent of sodium reabsorption, several studies have shown that increased
urinary salt excretion is associated with an increase in urinary cystine concentration
[15]. In a study in five children with cystinuria, the urinary cystine excretion was
measured after a week on an unrestricted sodium diet and compared to the urinary

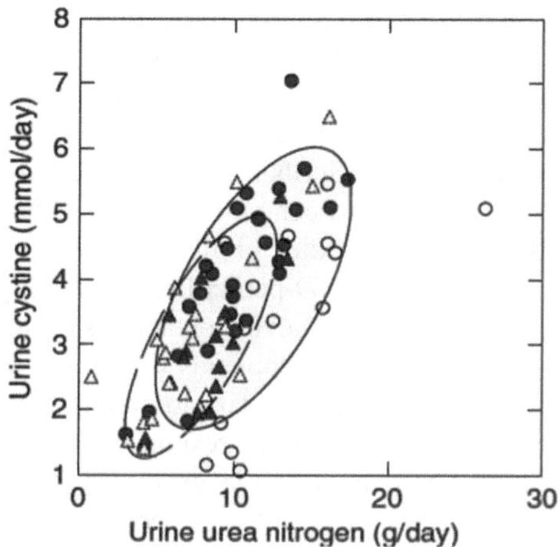

**Fig. 8.2** Increasing 24-h urine urea nitrogen was independently and strongly associated with increasing cystine excretion. *Circles*: men; *triangles*: women; *open symbols*: no thiol drugs; *closed symbols*: with thiols. *Ellipses* enclose 1 standard deviation from the mean; *solid line*: men; *broken line*: women. (Reproduced with permission from [13])



cystine excretion after a week on a sodium-restricted diet. They showed a marked reduction in urinary cystine excretion during the period of sodium restriction compared to that of unrestricted sodium, without a change in urine volume [16]. The pathophysiology remains to be elucidated; however, given its favorable effect salt restriction remains one of the mainstays of therapy. It is important to point out that although dietary protein and sodium intake have been clearly shown to increase cystine excretion, no trial has ever demonstrated that these dietary modifications are associated with reduced stone events. Nonetheless, we routinely prescribe them to our patients.

When patients with cystinuria are refractory to management with fluid therapy, alkali therapy, and dietary modifications, medication therapy with CBTDs is considered. Drugs containing a thiol group (-SH) are used to decrease excretion of cystine in the insoluble form. The drugs work by reducing the disulfide bond in cystine to yield two molecules of cysteine bound by the drugs' thiol groups to form soluble drug-cysteine complexes. The first such drug to be approved for use was D-penicillamine, although its use has been limited by a number of side effects associated with it. Tiopronin (or alpha-mercaptopropionylglycine) was later approved for use and although it was found to have similar side effects, the incidence of those side effects appeared to be decreased in comparison. Although the angiotensin-converting enzyme inhibitor captopril contains a thiol group and has also been used, its excretion in the urine is not sufficient to be effective in combining with urinary cystine.

Penicillamine was introduced as a therapy for cystinuria in 1963 [17]. Several small cohort studies showed that *D*-penicillamine effectively decreased the urinary excretion of cystine in patients with cystinuria, and even resulted in dissolution of stones in some cases [18, 19]. However, none of these studies had a control group for comparison, and most of the studies did not look at the effect on stone formation, so the true efficacy of the medication is still not known.

Tiopronin has also been used in the treatment of cystinuria since the 1970s [20]. Since its approval by FDA in 1986, there have been multiple small case series of patients treated with tiopronin that conclude that the medication is effective in decreasing the number of stone events. However, in most of the studies, the comparison is made to the same group of patients in the pretreatment period off medication, based on historical data alone [21, 22]. Although both *D*-penicillamine and tiopronin are often prescribed to cystinuric patients refractory to conservative management, there have been no randomized controlled trials of CBTDs to compare their efficacy to fluids, diet, or alkali.

The use of both *D*-penicillamine and tiopronin are limited by a number of side effects. The reported adverse reactions include allergy, fever, rash, nausea, vomiting, diarrhea, ageusia, cytopenias (including anemia, thrombocytopenia, and leukopenia), proteinuria (secondary to membranous nephropathy), elevated liver enzymes, and various autoimmune responses (systemic lupus erythematosis-like syndromes, polymyositis, myasthenia gravis, Goodpasture's syndrome, and thyroiditis). Although initially thought to be secondary to penicillamine itself, it is now recognized that the sulfhydryl group is responsible for these untoward effects, which are now considered a class effect [23]. The redox cycling that occurs between the thiol and the disulfide produces free radicals and "active oxygen" species that are believed to be responsible for the toxic effects of these compounds [24]. The reactions to the drugs are idiosyncratic and not necessarily dose related. As a result, a reaction to *D*-penicillamine does not necessarily predict that a reaction to tiopronin will occur [23]. Observational studies have also shown that withdrawal of the drug results in cessation of the side effect, and subsequent reinitiation of the drug at a lower dose is typically well tolerated [19]. As a result, desensitization protocols can be successful in reducing side effects in patients who have difficulty tolerating the drugs.

Overall, tiopronin has been found to be associated with fewer overall side effects than *D*-penicillamine, so it is usually the first-line drug of choice today. One study compared the rate of side effects between the two drugs in 49 patients who had been treated with *D*-penicillamine in the past [25]. It found that although adverse effects to tiopronin were still relatively frequent, with 30.6 % of subjects stopping therapy due to the adverse effects, it was a lower incidence compared to the prior treatment with *D*-penicillamine (in which 69.4 % of patients stopped therapy due to adverse effects). The study also showed that tiopronin was as effective as *D*-penicillamine at lowering urinary cystine excretion and more effective at preventing stone formation, with fewer stone events per year in the years they followed the patients on tiopronin compared to the historical control of stone events per year while on *D*-penicillamine. They attributed the increase in success of therapy with tiopronin compared to *D*-penicillamine to the increase in compliance in the setting of fewer adverse reactions [25].

A new alternative approach to prevention of recurrent nephrolithiasis is based on crystal growth inhibition. Ward and his lab at NYU are using atomic force microscopy (AFM) to visualize the early stages of organic crystal formation in liquids, including the nucleation events and topographic features that play a role in crystal formation [26]. Through this technique, they can also quantify the velocity of growth of a crystal, which allows them to study the effects of varying conditions, such as the presence of an inhibitor, on crystal formation. Through these studies of the structure and crystal formation of L-cystine in vitro, they were able to identify potential inhibitors of growth. The two most promising molecules they tested to date are L-cystine dimethyl ester (L-CDME) and L-cystine methyl ester (L-CME). They are structural mimics of cystine in which either one carboxyl group (in the case of L-CME) or two carboxyl groups (in L-CDME) are replaced by a methyl ester group. When added to L-cystine in vitro, these molecules were found to interfere with the formation of crystals, as seen by a roughening of the edges of the otherwise smooth hexagonal crystal structures that usually form in their absence. The velocity of crystal formation is also decreased by the inhibitors with an increasing effect as the concentration of inhibitor increases (until a certain concentration is reached).

One potential limitation of the molecules in therapeutic use is the potential for toxicity. Incubation of LLC-PK1 cells, a model for proximal tubule cells, with CDME, leads to the accumulation of cystine intracellularly, specifically within lysosomes [27]. Lysosomal accumulation of cystine also occurs in the autosomal recessive disease cystinosis, as a result of abnormal cystine transport. Clinically, this manifests as Fanconi's syndrome and even renal failure. The dose of the inhibitor would therefore have to prove to be effective at doses lower than those which cause this adverse effect. In vitro studies suggest that it is in fact potent enough to be effective without causing this adverse effect. Studies are now underway in Slc3a1 knockout mice to examine the inhibitor's ability to prevent formation of cystine stones as well as its side effects [28]. Although there is much work to be done on safety and efficacy, this body of work holds promise as a potential new therapeutic target in the future.

**Acknowledgments** We gratefully acknowledge the support of the Rare Kidney Stone Consortium (U54KD083908), a part of Rare Diseases Clinical Research Network (RDCRN), funded by the NIDDK and National Center For Advancing Translational Sciences (NCATS).

**Disclosures** No external funding sources contributed to this study. Goldfarb is a consultant for Takeda, Keryx; a CME speaker for Quintiles, Mission; owner of Ravine Group; and has received funding from NIDDK, ORDR.

# References

1. Chillarón J, Font-Llitjós M, Fort J, Zorzano A, Goldfarb DS, Nunes V, et al. Pathophysiology and treatment of cystinuria. Nat Rev Nephrol. 2010 Jul;6:424–34.
2. Segal S, Thier SO. Cystinuria. In: Scriver CR, Beaudet AL, Sly WS, Valle D, Editors. The metabolic basis of inherited disease. 6th edn. New York: McGraw-Hill; 1989. pp. 2479–96.
3. Della Strologo L, Pras E, Pontisilli C, Beccia E, Ricci-Barbini V, de Sanctis L, et al. Comparison between SLC3A1 and SLC7A9 cystinuria patients and carriers—a need for a new classification system. J Am Soc Nephrol. 2002 Oct;13(10):2547–53.
4. Gucev Z, Ristoska-Bojkovska N, Popovska-Jankovic K, Sukarova-Stefanovska E, Tasic V, Plaseska-Karanfilska D, et al. Cystinuria AA (B): Digenic inheritance with three mutations in two cystinuria genes. J Genet. 2011 Apr; 90(1):157–9.
5. Nakagawa Y, Asplin JR, Goldfarb DS, Parks JH, Coe FL. Clinical use of cystine supersaturation measurements. J Urol. 2000 Nov;164(5):1481–5.

6. Birwé H, Hesse A. High-performance liquid chromatographic determination of urinary cysteine and cystine. Clin Chim Acta. 1991 May;199(1):33–42.

7. Coe FL, Clark C, Parks JH, Asplin JR. Solid phase assay of urine cystine supersaturation in the presence of cystine binding drugs. J Urol. 2001 Aug;166(2):688–93.

8. Rule AD, Krambeck AE, Lieske JC. Chronic kidney disease in kidney stone formers. Clin J Am Soc Nephrol. 2011 Aug;6(8):2069–75.

9. Worcester EM, Parks JM, Evan AP, Coe FL. Renal function in patients with nephrolithiasis. J Urol. 2006 Aug;176(2):600–3.

10. Assimos DG, Leslie SW, Ng C, Streem SB, Hart LJ. The impact of cystinuria on renal function. J Urol. 2002 Jul;168(1):27–30.

11. Milliner D, Goldfarb DS, Beara-Lasic L, Edvardsson V, Bergstralh E, Lieske JC, et al. E19 Kidney function in genetic stone formers. Eur Urol Suppl 2013;12(3):36.

12. Dent CE, Senior B. Studies on the treatment of cystinuria. Br J Urol. 1955 Dec;27(4):317–32.

13. Goldfarb DS, Coe FC, Asplin JR. Urinary cystine excretion and capacity in patients with cystinuria. Kidney Int. 2006 Mar;69(6):1041–7.

14. Rodman JS, Blackburn P, Williams JJ, Brown A, Pospischil MA, Peterson CM. The effect of dietary protein on cystine excretion in patients with cystinuria. Clin Nephrol. 1984 Dec;22(6):273–8.

15. Jaeger P, Portmann L, Saunders A, Rosenberg LE, Their SO. Anticysinuric effects of glutamine and dietary sodium restriction. N Engl J Med. 1986 Oct 30;315(18):1120–3.

16. Rodríguez LM, Santos F, Málaga S, Martínez V. Effect of a low sodium diet on urinary elimination of cystine in cystinuric children. Nephron. 1995;71(4):416–8.

17. Crawhall JC, Scowen EF, Watts RW. Effect of peniciallamine of cystinuria. Br Med J. 1963 Mar 2;1(5330):588–90.

18. McDonald WB, Fellers FX. Penicillamine in the treatment of patients with cystinuria. J Am Med Assoc. 1966;197(6):396–402.

19. Dahlberg PJ, van den Berg CJ, Kurtz SB, Wilson DM, Smith LH. Clinical features and management of cystinuria. Mayo Clin Proc. 1977 Sep;52(9):533–42.

20. Remien A, Kallistratos G, Burchardt P. Treatment of cystinuria with Thiola. Eur Urol. 1975;1(5):227–8.

21. Barbey F, Joly D, Rieu P, Méjean A, Daudon M, Jungers P. Medical treatment of cystinuria: Critical appraisal of long-term results. J Urol. 2000 May;163(5):1419–23.

22. Della Stologo L, Laurenzi C, Legato A, Pastore A. Cystinuria in children and young adults: success in measuring free-cystine urine levels. Pediatr Nephrol. 2007 Nov; 22(11):1869–73.

23. Jaffe IA. Adverse effects profile of sulhydryl compounds in man. Am J Med. 1986 Mar;80(3):471–6.

24. Munday R. Toxicity of thiol and disulfides: Involvement of free radical species. Free Radic Biol Med. 1989;7(6):659–73.

25. Pak CY, Fuller C, Sakhaee K, Zerwekh JE, Adams BV. Management of cystine nephrolithiasis with alpha-mercaptopropionylglycine. J Urol. 1986 Nov;136(5):1003–8.

26. Rimer JD, An Z, Zhu Z, Lee MH, Goldfarb DS, Wesson JA, Ward MD. Crystal growth inhibitors for the prevention of L-cystine kidney stones through molecular design. Science. 2010 Oct;330(6002):337–41.

27. Moran A., Ben-Nun A, Potashnik R, Bashan N. Renal cells in culture as a model for cystinosis. J Basic Clin Physiol Pharmacol. 1990 Jan–Dec;1(1–4):357–72.

28. Sahota A, Yang M, Shikhel S, et al. Tailored inhibition of cystine stone formation as a therapy for cystinuria. J Inherit Metab Dis. 2012;35(S1):S27.

# Chapter 9
# Potassium Citrate and Calcium Stones: Benefit or Risk?

Ramy F. Youssef, Glenn M. Preminger and Michael E. Lipkin

## Background

The prevalence and incidence of nephrolithiasis is increasing worldwide [1]. The prevalence of nephrolithiasis has significantly increased in the USA from 3.8 % in 1980 to 9.8 % in 2010 [2]. Dietary and lifestyle changes may represent key factors responsible for this increase [1–3]. The lifetime prevalence of nephrolithiasis is approximately 10–13 % for adult men and 5–7 % for adult women, and the incidence is highest in the working population between 20 and 60 years [4,5]. The annual medical expenditures for the management of nephrolithiasis were estimated at US\$ 2.1 billion in 2000, representing a 50 % increase compared to 1994 [4,5]. An increase in the overall expenditures related to nephrolithiasis is expected [3].

The cost benefit of medical therapy for prevention of stone recurrence has been questioned [4–9]. Despite the higher cost; medical therapy may be more effective than conservative measures in reducing stone recurrence [6,10–13]. Remission rates under directed medical therapy reach as high as 90 % [14,15]. A meta-analysis of randomized trials demonstrated a 22.6 % risk reduction in recurrence rates with initiation of medical therapy and dietary management [16]. Appropriate medical treatment after surgical management (shock wave lithotripsy, ureteroscopy, and percutaneous nephrolithotomy) can inhibit new stone formation or growth of residual stone fragments in both adults and children [13,17,18].

Directed medical therapy based on metabolic evaluation is often instituted in patients with high risk of stone recurrence [6]. These patients include those with a strong family history of stones, those with intestinal disorders/chronic diarrhea, gout, bone disease, urinary tract abnormalities, children with nephrolithiasis, and patients with a solitary kidney or severe medical comorbidities. Metabolic evaluation and appropriate medical therapy should be considered in the majority of patients

M. E. Lipkin (✉) · R. F. Youssef · G. M. Preminger
Comprehensive Kidney Stone Center, Urology Division, Surgery Department,
Duke University Medical Center, 200 Trent Drive, Durham, NC 27710, USA
e-mail: michael.lipkin@duke.edu

M. S. Pearle, S. Y. Nakada (eds.), *Practical Controversies in Medical Management
of Stone Disease,* DOI 10.1007/978-1-4614-9575-8_9,
© Springer Science+Business Media New York 2014

**Table 9.1** Classification and incidence of metabolic diagnoses in patients with nephrolithiasis

|  | Sole occurrence | Combined occurrence |
| --- | --- | --- |
| Hypercalciuria | 20–30% | 40–60% |
| Hyperuricosuria | 10% | 40% |
| Hyperoxaluria | 10% | 50% |
| Hypocitraturia | 10–20% | 40–60% |
| Hypomagnesiuria | 5% | 10% |
| Gouty diathesis | 5–15% | 15–30% |
| Cystinuria | <1% | <1% |
| Infection stones | 1% | 5% |
| Low urine volume | 10% | 50% |

following any form of surgical stone removal, to prevent potential problems of residual stone growth or new stone formation. Calcium-based stones represent over 80% of the stone compositions encountered, with calcium oxalate monohydrate and calcium oxalate dihydrate each accounting for 40–60%. Calcium phosphate is less frequently encountered and accounts for 20–40% of stones analyzed [19]. Patients with calcium-based stones may be diagnosed with multiple metabolic abnormalities including hypercalcuria, hypocitraturia, hyperoxaluria, gouty diasthesis, hypomagnesuria, and low urine volumes. Table 9.1 demonstrates different metabolic diagnoses in stone formers.

This chapter will focus on the benefits and risks of potassium citrate as a medical treatment for the prevention of nephrolithiasis and its role in the treatment of different metabolic abnormalities.

## Mechanism of Action of Potassium Citrate

Potassium citrate is an oral alkalinizing agent that has been the mainstay of medical treatment for nephrolithiasis in the last three decades. Nearly all the supplementary citrate is absorbed from the gastrointestinal tract (GI tract), and the vast majority of this citrate load is metabolized by the liver to bicarbonate producing an alkaline load. The small portion of citrate that bypasses the liver passes into the serum and is excreted by the kidney. Importantly, pH impacts the citrate level in urine. As urinary pH increases, renal citrate production increases and tubular citrate reabsorption decreases [20,21]. Thus, potassium citrate increases urinary citrate mainly by modifying renal handling of citrate, rather than increasing the filtered load of citrate. It is important to note that citrate has a higher impact on urinary citrate than bicarbonate. The increase in urinary pH also decreases calcium ion activity by increasing calcium complexation to dissociated anions. The rise in urinary pH also increases the ionization of uric acid to the more soluble urate ion. Potassium citrate inhibits crystallization of stone-forming salts (calcium oxalate, calcium phosphate, and uric acid) [15,22]. These changes lead to decreased saturation of calcium oxalate. However, potassium citrate may not alter the urinary saturation of calcium phosphate,

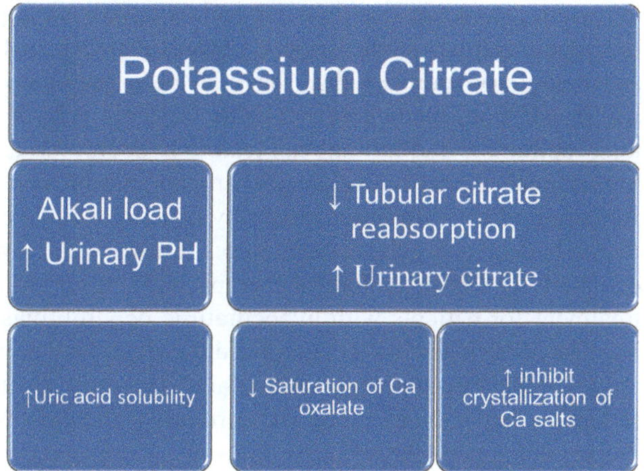


**Fig. 9.1** Physicochemical actions of potassium citrate

since the effect of increased citrate complexation of calcium is opposed by the rise in pH-dependent dissociation of phosphate. Figure 9.1 explains the physicochemical actions of potassium citrate.

In summary, potassium citrate increases urinary citrate and pH, decreases urinary calcium and calcium oxalate saturation, increases urinary uric acid concentration but also increases urinary uric acid solubility and has nearly no change on urinary oxalate or sulfate.

## Indications for Potassium Citrate

Potassium citrate has been successfully used in medical management of patients with nephrolithiasis with the following conditions:

1. Hypocitraturic nephrolithiasis of any etiology
2. Hypercalcuric patients in conjunction with thiazides
3. Renal tubular acidosis (RTA)
4. Chronic diarrheal syndromes
5. Gouty diathesis associated with uric acid stones or calcium oxalate stones

### *Potassium Citrate in Hypocitraturia*

Hypocitraturia, is a common metabolic abnormality which may be detected in up to 10 % as a solitary abnormality and up to 63 % as a mixed abnormality among patients with nephrolithiasis [23]. The definition of hypocitraturia might vary in different laboratories. We define normal urinary citrate as >450 mg/day in men and >550 mg/day in women in our current clinical practice. Hypocitraturia can be idiopathic. However, multiple risk factors have been implicated in the pathogenesis of hypocitraturia in stone formers. Chronic diarrhea, distal RTA, metabolic acidosis, and medullary sponge kidney have all been implicated as causes of hypocitraturia. In addition, medications such as carbonic anhydrase inhibitors; ACE inhibitors; topiramate and lithium can lead to hypocitraturia. Dietary factors including a high animal protein intake are also among possible causes [21]. Citrate inhibits the formation of calcium-based stones by forming soluble complexes with calcium, effectively decreasing the concentration of urinary calcium available to nucleate with oxalate [24]. Pharmacological therapy with citrate salts has been the mainstay of treatment for patients with hypocitraturic nephrolithiasis in the last three decades because of both its citrate content and the alkali load delivered to the kidneys. There are several citrate supplements available. However, potassium citrate remains a better option than sodium citrate and currently is the most commonly prescribed citrate preparation since 1980s [22,25–27].

The long-term effects of potassium-citrate therapy were examined in 89 patients with hypocitraturic calcium or uric acid nephrolithiasis in a nonrandomized, non-placebo-controlled clinical study. The dose of potassium citrate ranged from 30 to 100 mEq per day, and usually 20 mEq was administered orally three times daily. Patients were followed in an outpatient setting every 4 months during treatment and were studied over a period up to 4.33 years. Concomitant therapy (with thiazide or allopurinol) was allowed when indicated. Potassium citrate was associated with a sustained increase in urinary citrate from subnormal values to normal values (400–700 mg/day), and a sustained increase in urinary pH from 5.6 to 6.0 to approximately 6.5. No substantial or significant changes occurred in urinary uric acid, oxalate, sodium or phosphorus levels, or total volume. Owing to these physiological changes, uric acid solubility increased, urinary saturation of calcium oxalate decreased, and the propensity for spontaneous nucleation of calcium oxalate was reduced to normal. Moreover, stone formation decreased in 98 % of the patients, remission was observed in 80 %, and the need for surgical treatment due to newly formed stones was eliminated [25]. A randomized, double-blind trial assessing stone recurrence in patients with idiopathic hypocitraturia and calcium stones showed a significantly decreased stone recurrence rate in patients treated with potassium citrate compared with those who received placebo (20 vs. 73 %; $p < 0.05$) [15]. Another trial, which enrolled stone formers regardless of urine chemistry, also demonstrated a significantly decreased recurrence rate in patients who were given potassium magnesium citrate compared to placebo (remission rate 87 vs. 36 %, relative risk 0.06) [28]. Potassium citrate is the best medical option for patients with hypocitraturia, if there is no contraindication to its use (see contraindications and precautions section).

## Chronic Diarrhea

Patients with chronic diarrheal syndromes lose bicarbonate via the GI tract resulting in metabolic acidosis and impairment of citrate synthesis [29]. Besides hypocitraturia, patients with chronic diarrhea may have low urine volumes and hyperoxaluria as risk factors for stone formation. Potassium-citrate therapy in patients with hypocitraturia secondary to chronic diarrhea has been shown to reduce the stone formation rate and produce stone remission in 70% of patients [30]. The powder (liquid) form is preferable in cases of chronic diarrhea. Larger doses (60–120 mEq) might be needed and should be divided in three to four doses as it has relatively shorter duration of action [30]. Other treatment measures should include increasing fluid intake, limiting dietary oxalate, and adding calcium supplements, and perhaps pyridoxine (vitamin $B_6$) to control hyperoxaluria [31].

## Renal Tubular Acidosis

Distal RTA is associated with hypocitraturia, alkaline urine, acidosis, and hypokalemia. Young female patients who present with profound hypocitraturia, urinary pH>6.5, hypokalemic acidosis, and nephrocalcinosis often have this diagnosis. The effects of potassium citrate in a nonrandomized, nonplacebo-controlled clinical study of five men and four women with incomplete distal RTA with calcium oxalate/calcium phosphate nephrolithiasis were studied. The study included patients with a history of surgical removal of stones or stone passage during the last 3 years prior to initiation of potassium-citrate therapy. All patients started treatment with 60–80 mEq potassium citrate daily in three or four divided doses. Patients were given dietary recommendations including sodium-restricted diet (100 mEq/day) and reduction of oxalate intake (limited intake of nuts, dark roughage, chocolate, and tea). Patients with hypercalciuria were advised to moderately restrict calcium intake (400–800 mg/day). Potassium-citrate therapy was associated with inhibition of new stone formation in patients with distal tubular acidosis. Three of the nine patients continued to pass stones during the treatment phase, but at a significantly reduced rate. The stone-remission rate was 67%. All patients had a reduced stone formation rate. Over the first 2 years of treatment, the on-treatment stone formation rate was reduced from $13\pm27$ to $1\pm2$ per year [26]. Potassium citrate can correct metabolic acidosis and hypokalemia in patients with distal RTA. Moreover, it restores normal urinary-citrate levels although larger doses of potassium citrate may be required [26].

Another study evaluating long-term treatment with potassium citrate in patients with medullary sponge kidney, a condition associated with renal tubular acidosis in up to 40% of cases, found a significant rise in urinary citrate and decrease in urinary calcium. Potassium citrate led to dramatic reduction in stone related events (from 0.58 to 0.1 stones/year/patient) [10].

It is to be noted that in patients with severe RTA or chronic diarrheal syndrome where urinary citrate may be very low (<100 mg/day), potassium citrate may be relatively ineffective in raising urinary citrate and a higher dose may therefore be required to produce a satisfactory alkali citraturic response. In patients with renal tubular acidosis in whom urinary pH may be high, potassium citrate produces a relatively small rise in urinary pH. If there is a significant rise in urinary pH consideration should be made for dose reduction or alternative therapy as there may be an increased risk of calcium phosphate stone formation.

## *Thiazide-Induced Hypocitraturia*

Thiazide therapy may induce hypokalemia and hypocitraturia; therefore, potassium citrate is commonly administered in conjunction with thiazides used for the treatment of hypercalciuria [32,33]. A study combining thiazides and potassium citrate with dietary modifications in 28 patients with type I absorptive hypercalciuria found a significant decrease in urinary calcium, no change in urinary oxalate, and an increase in urinary pH and citrate; urinary saturation of calcium oxalate significantly decreased by 46%. The stone-formation rate decreased significantly from 2.94 to 0.05/year ($p < 0.001$) [33].

In our practice, potassium citrate is used in conjunction with thiazide therapy for medical prophylaxis in patients with absorptive hypercalciuria type I. Serum electrolytes and kidney function are routinely checked 2 weeks after initiation of treatment. The majority of these patients are maintained on chlorthalidone 25 mg once daily and potassium citrate 20–30 mEq bid with meals. The doses can be adjusted according to follow-up metabolic profiles.

## *Gouty Diathesis Associated with Uric Acid Stones or Calcium Oxalate Stones*

Potassium citrate is used for treatment in patients with gouty diathesis (low urinary pH < 5.5), whether it is sole metabolic abnormality or with other abnormalities. A long-term nonrandomized, nonplacebo-controlled clinical trial with 18 adult patients with uric acid lithiasis (six with pure uric acid stones and 12 with mixed stones containing both calcium and uric acid) received long-term treatment of potassium citrate for up to 5.33 years. Eleven of the 18 patients received potassium citrate alone. Six of the seven other patients also received allopurinol for hyperuricemia with gouty arthritis, symptomatic hyperuricemia, or hyperuricosuria. One patient also received hydrochlorothiazide because of unclassified hypercalciuria. The main inclusion criterion was a history of stone passage or surgical removal of stones during the 3 years prior to initiation of potassium-citrate therapy. All patients received potassium citrate at a dosage of 30–80 mEq/day in three to four divided doses and were followed every 4 months for up to 5 years. While on potassium-citrate treatment, urinary pH rose significantly from $5.3 \pm 0.3$ to within normal limits (6.2–6.5). Urinary citrate rose from $503 \pm 225$ mg/day to 852 to 998 mg/day. Urinary saturation of calcium oxalate significantly declined with potassium-citrate treatment. New stone-formation rate declined from 1.2 stones/year to 0.01 stones/year ($p < 0.001$). Remission was observed in 94% of patients, and the group stone formation rate declined by >99% as only one stone was formed in the entire group of 18 patients [34].

Potassium citrate is our preferred medical treatment for stone formers with gouty diathesis or low urinary pH. Potassium citrate is the preferred primary treatment for the prevention of recurrent uric acid stones. Sodium bicarbonate can serve as an alternative, when there is contraindication or intolerability for use of potassium citrate.

## Effectiveness of Long-term Potassium-Citrate Therapy

Three decades of clinical use of potassium citrate as a medical prophylaxis in stone formers had confirmed its effectiveness and safety. A retrospective evaluation of 503 patients who received potassium citrate for a mean duration of 41 months (range 6–168) was performed. Changes in urinary profiles included increased urinary pH (5.90–6.46, $p < 0.0001$) and increased urinary citrate (470–700 mg/day, $p < 0.0001$) and were noted as soon as 6 months after the onset of therapy. The stone-formation rate also significantly decreased after the initiation of potassium citrate from 1.89 to 0.46 stones per year ($p < 0.0001$). There was a 68 % remission rate and a 93 % decrease in the stone-formation rate. The changes in urinary metabolic profiles were sustained for as long as 14 years of treatment. These results confirmed the long-term effectiveness of potassium-citrate therapy in patients with recurrent nephrolithiasis [12].

## Effect of Potassium-Citrate Therapy on Bone

Potassium citrate may avert age-dependent bone loss. Mineral bone density was studied in a group of 16 men and five women with stones taking potassium citrate from 11 to 120 months. Bone mineral density increased significantly by 3.1 % over a mean duration of 44 months. Urinary pH, citrate, and potassium increased significantly during treatment but urinary calcium did not change [35].

Another two-phase crossover randomized trial compared potassium calcium citrate to placebo in preventing metabolic abnormalities in 24 patients undergoing Roux-en-Y gastric bypass surgery. Potassium calcium citrate was found to inhibit bone resorption by providing bioavailable calcium, reduced the urinary saturation of uric acid, and increased the inhibitor activity against calcium oxalate agglomeration by providing alkali that increased urinary pH and citrate [36]. A third study combining dietary efforts with combined treatment with thiazides and potassium citrate for patients with type I absorptive hypercalciuria, found not only improvement in metabolic profiles and stone-formation rate but also bone mineral density increased significantly by 5.7 % compared to normal peak value, and by 7.1 % compared with normal age and gender-matched value [33].

## Impact of Potassium Citrate on Residual Stones After Surgical Treatment

The beneficial effect of medical therapies after percutaneous nephrolithotomy or shock wave lithotripsy was demonstrated in multiple studies. The proper establishment of medical therapy after surgical management may result in stabilization of stone disease and prevention of the need for further surgical procedures for stone removal. These beneficial effects were noticed in patients with or without residual stone fragments after surgical management or shock wave lithotripsy [11,13,17,18,37–39].

The effect of selective medical therapy after percutaneous nephrolithotomy was evaluated in 70 patients. Medical therapy significantly decreased stone-formation rates in stone-free patients (0.67 vs. 0.02 stones/patient/year) and patients with residual fragments (0.67 vs. 0.02 stones/patient/year, $p<0.0001$). Remission increased in stone-free and residual fragment groups (87 and 77%) when compared to the same groups without medical therapy (29 and 21%, $p<0.0001$) [13].

Similar findings were identified after shock wave lithotripsy. A prospective, randomized trial evaluated the efficacy of potassium-citrate therapy in reducing stone recurrence or regrowth in patients undergoing shockwave lithotripsy for lower calyceal stones. A total of 90 patients, including 56 stone-free patients and 34 patients with residual fragments, were randomized to receive either 60 mEq of potassium citrate daily or no treatment 4 weeks after undergoing shockwave lithotripsy for lower pole stones. Potassium citrate reduced the rate of stone recurrence or stone growth in stone-free patients or those with residual fragments after shockwave lithotripsy. In stone-free patients, no stone recurrences occurred in those treated with potassium citrate, while 28.5% of control patients experienced recurrence. In patients with residual fragments, 45.5% demonstrated clearance of the fragments during follow-up, and the remaining 54.5% of patients showed no stone growth or recurrence. In the control group, however, only 12.5% of patients cleared their residual fragments, 25% of patients showed no change in the size of the stones, and 62% demonstrated stone growth. Of additional interest, potassium citrate also apparently facilitated the discharge of residual lower pole fragments in patients with residual stones [17]. The beneficial effect of potassium-citrate therapy after shockwave lithotripsy was not only observed in adults, but also in children [18].

We recommend directed medical therapy based on metabolic evaluation after surgical management of stone disease. This policy decreases stone recurrence in stone-free patients. Moreover, it helps stone remission in patients with residual fragments and decreases the stone-related events and future need for surgery.

## Dose Adjustments and Follow-up

The goal for use of potassium citrate is to correct hypocitraturia in calcium-based stones and maintain urinary pH between 6 and 6.5 in stone formers with low urinary pH. The starting dose usually ranges between 30 and 60 mEq daily; divided into two or three times with meals; depending on the severity of hypocitraturia. Caution should be used in patients with renal insufficiency and a lower starting dose should be instituted. Patients are instructed to start therapy gradually with meals to increase tolerability and avoid side effects. Serum electrolytes and creatinine are monitored before and 2–3 weeks after therapy, especially in patients at risk of hyperkalemia. Treatment should be discontinued in the presence of hyperkalemia or significant rise of serum creatinine. Metabolic profiles based on 24-h urine collections are re-checked initially in a few months (usually 4 months) to adjust the dose according to urinary pH and changes noted in the metabolic profile. The follow-up intervals may increase later gradually to 6 months then yearly intervals.

## Does Potassium Citrate Increase the Risk of CaP Stones?

There has been concern that potassium citrate's effect of increasing urinary pH may potentially promote the precipitation of calcium phosphate crystals in susceptible individuals. Urine pH and CaP supersaturaion were found to increase in proportion to average percent of CaP in the stone composition [40]. However, the same study did not find a difference in stone-relapse rates between different stone compositions (CaP and CaOx) and both did well with medical prevention, including potassium citrate. While previous studies including randomized, controlled trials confirmed short-term and long-term effectiveness of potassium-citrate therapy on urinary profiles and recurrent stone formation, there are sparse data on the risk of calcium phosphate stones forming after introduction of alkali therapy. Acidic urine with low pH predisposes to calcium stones as well as uric acid stones. Alkalinzing agents like potassium citrate have been used to raise urine pH and prevent stone formation. A balance is needed as too high urinary pH (urine pH > 7) might lead to formation of calcium phosphate stones. In our clinical practice, patients are followed up with 24-h urine collections to adjust treatment doses based on the changes in metabolic profiles and urinary pH. In patients who have an excessive rise in urinary pH (greater than 7), the dose of potassium citrate should be reduced. As such, the risk of development of calcium phosphate stones is minimized.

## Adverse Reactions and Compliance

One of the concerns about medical therapy for prevention of stone growth/recurrence is patient compliance. Some patients do not take their medication every day and might be more comfortable trying dietary modifications. In a survey of 100 patients undergoing intervention for nephrolithiasis at a Swedish center, 95 patients were motivated to change their dietary habits, whereas only 71 desired pharmacologic treatment. Interest in medical therapy was the lowest-reported preference, below interest in collecting a second 24-h urine sample [41]. Another study that surveyed both first time and recurrent stone formers found that patients in both groups expressed a preference for dietary intervention over pharmacotherapy [42]. A third study that looked at long-term follow-up of stone formers who were treated with

                                                              

**Table 9.2** Comparison between tablet and liquid forms of pottasium citrate

|                     | Liquid   | Tablets    |
| ------------------- | -------- | ---------- |
| Minor Gl complaints | +        | ++         |
| Gastric erosions    | 0        | 0/+        |
| Convenience         | +        | +++        |
| Citraturic action   | ++       | +++        |
| Half-life           | Short    | Prolonged  |
| Dose schedule       | tid/qid  | bid/tid    |

low doses of sodium potassium citrate, only 62 % consistently took the medication [43]. The problems with compliance are poorly reported in the literature, but some reasons cited are high cost, gastrointestinal side effects (abdominal pain, nausea, vomiting, diarrhea), bad taste, and inconvenience of bid or tid dosing [23,44,45]. Gastrointestinal side effects were reported in 10 % of patients on potassium-citrate therapy [21,25,28]. The wax matrix component of the tablet might be secreted intact in stool, and patients should be reassured that the medication is being properly absorbed [46,47].

Potassium citrate is commonly used in the tablet form, however, a powder/liquid form might be more preferable in cases of chronic diarrhea or in patients who experience gastrointestinal upset. Table 9.2 includes the differences between both forms. Poor palatability may lead to poor compliance with the powder form of potassium citrate. One possible way to improve palatability and compliance is to add an artificial sweetener to the powder form. In a recent study, taste was judged to be significantly better in the Splenda + potassium citrate compared with potassium citrate alone. The 24-h citrate, K, and pH were significantly higher in the potassium citrate and potassium citrate + Splenda groups compared with baseline, but not significantly different from each other. Splenda significantly improves the palatability of potassium-citrate therapy and did not alter the beneficial effects of potassium citrate on 24-h urine citrate, K, or pH [45].

## Contraindications and Precautions

Despite the proven effectiveness and safety of potassium-citrate therapy in stone prophylaxis, it is not devoid of possible side effects. The first contraindication to the use of potassium citrate is in patients with hyperkalemia, as a further rise in serum potassium may produce cardiac arrest. This should be a concern in patients with chronic kidney disease, heart problems, or with intake of potassium-sparing diuretics. Potassium citrate should not be used when glomerular filtration rate is reduced (creatinine > 2.5 mg/dL).

Potassium citrate may irritate the GI tract and should not be used in patients with gastritis or peptic ulcer. If there is severe vomiting, abdominal pain, or gastrointestinal bleeding, potassium citrate should be discontinued immediately. Clinicians should think of alternatives to potassium citrate in patients in whom there is cause for arrest or delay in tablet passage through the GI tract, such as those suffering from delayed gastric emptying, esophageal compression, intestinal obstruction or stricture, or those taking anticholinergic medication.

## Dietary Alternatives and Adjuncts to Potassium-Citrate Therapy

While potassium-citrate therapy is the best option for prophylaxis of recurrent calcium nephrolithiasis in hypocitraturic stone formers, some patients prefer non-pharmacological intervention. Citrus juices are a known natural source of dietary citrate, and several studies have investigated their impact on urinary profiles [21,24,48–52].

Orange juice can increase urinary pH and citrate [51]. However, it may also increase urinary oxalate. It might be ineffective in decreasing urinary saturation of calcium oxalate [50]. Another study investigated the impact of orange, grapefruit, or apple juice on urinary profiles. An increase in pH and citrate excretion was observed with each of the three juices, but the decrease in relative supersaturation of calcium oxalate crystallization was significant only for grapefruit juice [51]. However, another study found an increase in urinary oxalate and citrate excretion with no change in the supersaturation of calcium oxalate, calcium phosphate, or uric acid [52]. Lemon juice appears to have the highest concentration of citrate of all citrus juices. It leads to an increase in urine volume and citrate, and a decrease in urinary calcium. Previous studies had shown that lemon juice is an inexpensive and well-tolerated dietary source of citrate that may improve patient compliance and be used as adjunctive therapy in patients with hypocitraturia [6,24,48,49,53]. An increase in urinary oxalate, a risk seen with orange juice administration, was not observed in patients on lemonade therapy [49]. Long-term lemonade therapy was able to decrease the stone formation rate from 1.00 to 0.13 stones per patient per year ($p < 0.05$) [49].

It should be noted that slow-release potassium citrate has a significantly greater citraturic response compared to lemonade therapy. The citraturic action of potassium citrate might be attributed to the combined effect of alkali load delivered by oxidation of citrate to bicarbonate and direct renal excretion of citrate [12,20–22,34,49]. In contrast, lemonade therapy does not deliver a urinary alkali load due to the low pH of lemon juice. Rather, it induces a citraturic response through the renal excretion of nonmetabolized citrate alone. Lemonade does not impact urine pH, so this treatment is not recommended for patient who would benefit from the alkali effect of potassium citrate [49,54]. Lemonade should be considered as adjunctive to potassium-citrate therapy or alternative in patients with poor compliance or who refuse medical therapy in presence of mild hypocitraturia.

## Future Directions and Potential New Indications for Potassium Citrate

### *Can Potassium-Citrate Therapy Facilitate Medical Expulsive Therapy?*

The role of combined potassium citrate and tamsulosin in the management of uric acid distal ureteral calculi was recently studied in 191 patients. The study was designed as a prospective, double-blind, randomized, controlled trial. The authors concluded that alkalization with potassium citrate combined with tamsulosin can increase the chances of spontaneous passage of radiolucent distal ureteral uric acid stones, especially those of 8–11 mm [55].

### *Potassium Citrate to Decrease the Risk of Stone Formation During Spaceflight*

Exposure to microgravity affects human physiology and results in changes in urinary chemistry during and after spaceflight, favoring an increased risk of renal stones. A study was done in 30 long duration spaceflight crew members. Crew members treated with potassium citrate had decreased urinary calcium excretion and maintained the calcium oxalate supersaturation risk at preflight levels compared to that in controls. Increased urinary pH in the treatment group decreased the risk of uric acid stones. Results from this investigation suggest that supplementation with potassium citrate may decrease the risk of renal-stone formation during and immediately after spaceflight [56].

## Conclusion

A multimodal approach with medical therapy, lifestyle changes, and dietary adjustments may be needed to control multiple or complex metabolic abnormalities in recurrent stone formers. Potassium-citrate therapy was proven effective when used with other medications and diet/lifestyle modifications in decreasing stone formation/recurrence rate. Potassium citrate can reverse the underlying physicochemical and physiological abnormalities implicated in stone formation. Moreover, it may overcome nonrenal complications and preserve bone in conditions like RTA. Potassium citrate is generally safe and considered free of serious side effects if used appropriately. Patients on medical therapy for nephrolithiasis should be followed up periodically to make sure they maintain normal metabolic profiles and minimize stone-related events.

# References


1. Romero V, Akpinar H, Assimos DG. Kidney stones: a global picture of prevalence, incidence, and associated risk factors. Rev Urol. 2010 Spring;12(2–3):e86–96. (PubMed PMID: 20811557. Pubmed Central PMCID: PMC2931286. Epub 2010/09/03. Eng).

2. Scales CD Jr., Smith AC, Hanley JM, Saigal CS. Prevalence of kidney stones in the United States. Eur Urol. 2012 Jul;62(1):160–5. (PubMed PMID: 22498635. Pubmed Central PMCID: PMC3362665. Epub 2012/04/14. Eng).

3. Brikowski TH, Lotan Y, Pearle MS. Climate-related increase in the prevalence of urolithiasis in the United States. Proc Nat Acad Sci U S A. 2008 Jul 15;105(28):9841–6. (PubMed PMID: 18626008. Pubmed Central PMCID: PMC2474527. Epub 2008/07/16. Eng).

4. Lotan Y, Pearle MS. Economics of stone management. Urol Cli North Am. 2007 Aug;34(3):443–53. (PubMed PMID: 17678993. Epub 2007/08/07. Eng).

5. Lotan Y, Pearle MS. Cost-effectiveness of primary prevention strategies for nephrolithiasis. J Urol. 2011 Aug;186(2):550–5. (PubMed PMID: 21683379. Epub 2011/06/21. Eng).

6. Lipkin M, Shah O. Medical therapy of stone disease: from prevention to promotion of passage options. Curr Urol Rep. 2009 Jan;10(1):29–34. (PubMed PMID: 19116093. Epub 2009/01/01. Eng).

7. Lotan Y. Economics and cost of care of stone disease. Adv Chronic Kidney Dis. 2009 Jan;16(1):5–10. (PubMed PMID: 19095200. Epub 2008/12/20. Eng).

8. Lotan Y, Cadeddu JA, Pearle MS. International comparison of cost effectiveness of medical management strategies for nephrolithiasis. Urol Res. 2005 Jun;33(3):223–30. (PubMed PMID: 15924256. Epub 2005/06/01. Eng).

9. Lotan Y, Cadeddu JA, Roerhborn CG, Pak CY, Pearle MS. Cost-effectiveness of medical management strategies for nephrolithiasis. J Urol. 2004 Dec;172(6 Pt 1):2275–81. (PubMed PMID: 15538248. Epub 2004/11/13. Eng).

10. Fabris A, Lupo A, Bernich P, Abaterusso C, Marchionna N, Nouvenne A et al. Long-term treatment with potassium citrate and renal stones in medullary sponge kidney. Clin J Am Soc Nephrol. 2010 Sep;5(9):1663–8. (PubMed PMID: 20576821. Pubmed Central PMCID: PMC2974409. Epub 2010/06/26. Eng).

11. Zilberman DE, Preminger GM. Long-term results of percutaneous nephrolithotomy: does prophylactic medical stone management make a difference? J Endourol. 2009 Oct;23(10):1773–6. (PubMed PMID: 19530951. Epub 2009/06/18. Eng).

12. Robinson MR, Leitao VA, Haleblian GE, Scales CD Jr, Chandrashekar A, Pierre SA et al. Impact of long-term potassium citrate therapy on urinary profiles and recurrent stone formation. J Urol. 2009 Mar;181(3):1145–50. (PubMed PMID: 19152932. Epub 2009/01/21. Eng).

13. Kang DE, Maloney MM, Haleblian GE, Springhart WP, Honeycutt EF, Eisenstein EL et al. Effect of medical management on recurrent stone formation following percutaneous nephrolithotomy. J Urol. 2007 May;177(5):1785–8. (discussion 8–9. PubMed PMID: 17437820. Epub 2007/04/18. Eng).

14. Delvecchio FC, Preminger GM. Medical management of stone disease. Curr Opin Urol. 2003 May;13(3):229–33. (PubMed PMID: 12692447. Epub 2003/04/15. Eng).

15. Barcelo P, Wuhl O, Servitge E, Rousaud A, Pak CY. Randomized double-blind study of potassium citrate in idiopathic hypocitraturic calcium nephrolithiasis. J Urol. 1993 Dec;150(6):1761–4. (PubMed PMID: 8230497. Epub 1993/12/01. Eng).

16. Pearle MS, Roehrborn CG, Pak CY. Meta-analysis of randomized trials for medical prevention of calcium oxalate nephrolithiasis. J Endourol. 1999 Nov;13(9):679–85. (PubMed PMID: 10608521. Epub 1999/12/23. Eng).

17. Soygur T, Akbay A, Kupeli S. Effect of potassium citrate therapy on stone recurrence and residual fragments after shockwave lithotripsy in lower caliceal calcium oxalate urolithiasis: a randomized controlled trial. J Endourol. 2002 Apr;16(3):149–52. (PubMed PMID: 12028622. Epub 2002/05/25. Eng).

18. Sarica K, Erturhan S, Yurtseven C, Yagci F. Effect of potassium citrate therapy on stone recurrence and regrowth after extracorporeal shockwave lithotripsy in children. J Endourol. 2006 Nov;20(11):875–9. (PubMed PMID: 17144854. Epub 2006/12/06. Eng).
19. Moe OW. Kidney stones: pathophysiology and medical management. Lancet. 2006 Jan 28;367(9507):333–44. (PubMed PMID: 16443041. Epub 2006/01/31. Eng).
20. Zuckerman JM, Assimos DG. Hypocitraturia: pathophysiology and medical management. Rev Urol. 2009 Summer;11(3):134–44. (PubMed PMID: 19918339. Pubmed Central PMCID: PMC2777061. Epub 2009/11/18. Eng).
21. Kurtz MP, Eisner BH. Dietary therapy for patients with hypocitraturic nephrolithiasis. Nat Rev Urol. 2011 Mar;8(3):146–52. (PubMed PMID: 21321574. Epub 2011/02/16. Eng).
22. Preminger GM, Harvey JA, Pak CY. Comparative efficacy of "specific" potassium citrate therapy versus conservative management in nephrolithiasis of mild to moderate severity. J Urol. 1985 Oct;134(4):658–61. (PubMed PMID: 3897582. Epub 1985/10/01. Eng).
23. Tracy CR, Pearle MS. Update on the medical management of stone disease. Curr Opin Urol. 2009 Mar;19(2):200–4. (PubMed PMID: 19188774. Epub 2009/02/04. Eng).
24. Seltzer MA, Low RK, McDonald M, Shami GS, Stoller ML. Dietary manipulation with lemonade to treat hypocitraturic calcium nephrolithiasis. J Urol. 1996 Sep;156(3):907–9. (PubMed PMID: 8709360. Epub 1996/09/01. Eng).
25. Pak CY, Fuller C, Sakhaee K, Preminger GM, Britton F. Long-term treatment of calcium nephrolithiasis with potassium citrate. J Urol. 1985 Jul;134(1):11–9. (PubMed PMID: 3892044. Epub 1985/07/01. Eng).
26. Preminger GM, Sakhaee K, Skurla C, Pak CY. Prevention of recurrent calcium stone formation with potassium citrate therapy in patients with distal renal tubular acidosis. J Urol. 1985 Jul;134(1):20–3. (PubMed PMID: 4009822. Epub 1985/07/01. Eng).
27. Preminger GM, Sakhaee K, Pak CY. Alkali action on the urinary crystallization of calcium salts: contrasting responses to sodium citrate and potassium citrate. J Urol. 1988 Feb;139(2):240–2. (PubMed PMID: 3339718. Epub 1988/02/01. Eng).
28. Ettinger B, Pak CY, Citron JT, Thomas C, Adams-Huet B, Vangessel A. Potassium-magnesium citrate is an effective prophylaxis against recurrent calcium oxalate nephrolithiasis. J Urol. 1997 Dec;158(6):2069–73. (PubMed PMID: 9366314. Epub 1997/11/20. Eng).
29. Rudman D, Dedonis JL, Fountain MT, Chandler JB, Gerron GG, Fleming GA et al. Hypocitraturia in patients with gastrointestinal malabsorption. N Engl J Med. 1980 Sep 18;303(12):657–61. (PubMed PMID: 7402252. Epub 1980/09/18. Eng).
30. Pak CY, Skurla C, Brinkley L, Sakhaee K. Augmentation of renal citrate excretion by oral potassium citrate administration: time course, dose frequency schedule, and dose-response relationship. J Clin Pharmacol. 1984 Jan;24(1):19–26.( PubMed PMID: 6707230. Epub 1984/01/01. Eng).
31. Ortiz-Alvarado O, Miyaoka R, Kriedberg C, Moeding A, Stessman M, Monga M. Pyridoxine and dietary counseling for the management of idiopathic hyperoxaluria in stone-forming patients. Urology. 2011 May;77(5):1054–8. (PubMed PMID: 21334732. Epub 2011/02/22. Eng).
32. Odvina CV, Preminger GM, Lindberg JS, Moe OW, Pak CY. Long-term combined treatment with thiazide and potassium citrate in nephrolithiasis does not lead to hypokalemia or hypochloremic metabolic alkalosis. Kidney Int. 2003 Jan;63(1):240–7. (PubMed PMID: 12472789. Epub 2002/12/11. Eng).
33. Pak CY, Heller HJ, Pearle MS, Odvina CV, Poindexter JR, Peterson RD. Prevention of stone formation and bone loss in absorptive hypercalciuria by combined dietary and pharmacological interventions. J Urol. 2003 Feb;169(2):465–9. (PubMed PMID: 12544288. Epub 2003/01/25. Eng).
34. Pak CY, Sakhaee K, Fuller C. Successful management of uric acid nephrolithiasis with potassium citrate. Kidney Int. 1986 Sep;30(3):422–8. (PubMed PMID: 3784284. Epub 1986/09/01. Eng).
35. Pak CY, Peterson RD, Poindexter J. Prevention of spinal bone loss by potassium citrate in cases of calcium urolithiasis. J Urol. 2002 Jul;168(1):31–4. (PubMed PMID: 12050486. Epub 2002/06/07. Eng).

36. Sakhaee K, Griffith C, Pak CY. Biochemical control of bone loss and stone-forming propensity by potassium-calcium citrate after bariatric surgery. Surg Obes Relat Dis. 2012 Jan-Feb;8(1):67–72. (PubMed PMID: 21703942. Epub 2011/06/28. Eng).

37. Lojanapiwat B, Tanthanuch M, Pripathanont C, Ratchanon S, Srinualnad S, Taweemonkongsap T et al. Alkaline citrate reduces stone recurrence and regrowth after shockwave lithotripsy and percutaneous nephrolithotomy. Int Braz J Urol. 2011 Sep-Oct;37(5):611–6. (PubMed PMID: 22099273. Epub 2011/11/22. Eng).

38. Fine JK, Pak CY, Preminger GM. Effect of medical management and residual fragments on recurrent stone formation following shock wave lithotripsy. J Urol. 1995 Jan;153(1):27–32. (discussion –3. PubMed PMID: 7966783. Epub 1995/01/01. Eng).

39. Cicerello E, Merlo F, Gambaro G, Maccatrozzo L, Fandella A, Baggio B et al. Effect of alkaline citrate therapy on clearance of residual renal stone fragments after extracorporeal shock wave lithotripsy in sterile calcium and infection nephrolithiasis patients. Journal Urol. 1994 Jan;151(1):5–9. (PubMed PMID: 8254832. Epub 1994/01/01. Eng).

40. Parks JH, Worcester EM, Coe FL, Evan AP, Lingeman JE. Clinical implications of abundant calcium phosphate in routinely analyzed kidney stones. Kidney Int. 2004 Aug;66(2):777–85. (PubMed PMID: 15253733. Epub 2004/07/16. Eng).

41. Tiselius HG. Patients' attitudes on how to deal with the risk of future stone recurrences. Urol Res. 2006 Aug;34(4):255–60. (PubMed PMID: 16642318. Epub 2006/04/28. Eng).

42. Grampsas SA, Moore M, Chandhoke PS. 10-year experience with extracorporeal shockwave lithotripsy in the state of Colorado. J Endourol. 2000 Nov;14(9):711–4. (PubMed PMID: 11110562. Epub 2000/12/08. Eng).

43. Jendle-Bengten C, Tiselius HG. Long-term follow-up of stone formers treated with a low dose of sodium potassium citrate. Scand J Urol Nephrol. 2000 Feb;34(1):36–41. (PubMed PMID: 10757268. Epub 2000/04/11. Eng).

44. Schwille PO, Herrmann U, Wolf C, Berger I, Meister R. Citrate and recurrent idiopathic calcium urolithiasis. A longitudinal pilot study on the metabolic effects of oral potassium citrate administered over the short-, medium- and long-term medication of male stone patients. Urol Res. 1992;20(2):145–55. (PubMed PMID: 1553790. Epub 1992/01/01. Eng).

45. Mechlin C, Kalorin C, Asplin J, White M. Splenda(R) improves tolerance of oral potassium citrate supplementation for prevention of stone formation: results of a randomized double-blind trial. J Endourol. 2011 Sep;25(9):1541–5. (PubMed PMID: 21815827. Epub 2011/08/06. Eng).

46. Gonzalez GB, Pak CY, Adams-Huet B, Taylor R, Bilhartz LE. Effect of potassium-magnesium citrate on upper gastrointestinal mucosa. Aliment Pharmacol Ther. 1998 Jan;12(1):105–10. (PubMed PMID: 9692708. Epub 1998/08/06. Eng).

47. Fegan J, Khan R, Poindexter J, Pak CY. Gastrointestinal citrate absorption in nephrolithiasis. J Urol. 1992 May;147(5):1212–4. (PubMed PMID: 1569651. Epub 1992/05/01. Eng).

48. Penniston KL, Steele TH, Nakada SY. Lemonade therapy increases urinary citrate and urine volumes in patients with recurrent calcium oxalate stone formation. Urology. 2007 Nov;70(5):856–60. (PubMed PMID: 17919696. Epub 2007/10/09. Eng).

49. Kang DE, Sur RL, Haleblian GE, Fitzsimons NJ, Borawski KM, Preminger GM. Long-term lemonade based dietary manipulation in patients with hypocitraturic nephrolithiasis. J Urol. 2007 Apr;177(4):1358–62. (discussion 62; quiz 591. PubMed PMID: 17382731. Epub 2007/03/27. Eng).

50. Wabner CL, Pak CY. Effect of orange juice consumption on urinary stone risk factors. J Urol. 1993 Jun;149(6):1405–8. (PubMed PMID: 8501777. Epub 1993/06/01. Eng).

51. Honow R, Laube N, Schneider A, Kessler T, Hesse A. Influence of grapefruit-, orange- and apple-juice consumption on urinary variables and risk of crystallization. Br J Nutr. 2003 Aug;90(2):295–300. (PubMed PMID: 12908889. Epub 2003/08/12. Eng).

52. Goldfarb DS, Asplin JR. Effect of grapefruit juice on urinary lithogenicity. J Urol. 2001 Jul;166(1):263–7. (PubMed PMID: 11435883. Epub 2001/07/04. Eng).

53. Aras B, Kalfazade N, Tugcu V, Kemahli E, Ozbay B, Polat H et al. Can lemon juice be an alternative to potassium citrate in the treatment of urinary calcium stones in patients with

hypocitraturia? A prospective randomized study. Urol Res. 2008 Dec;36(6):313–7. (PubMed PMID: 18946667. Epub 2008/10/24. Eng).

54. Sakhaee K, Alpern R, Poindexter J, Pak CY. Citraturic response to oral citric acid load. J Urol. 1992 Apr;147(4):975–6. (PubMed PMID: 1552616. Epub 1992/04/01. Eng).

55. El-Gamal O, El-Bendary M, Ragab M, Rasheed M. Role of combined use of potassium citrate and tamsulosin in the management of uric acid distal ureteral calculi. Urol Res. 2012 Jun;40(3):219–24. (PubMed PMID: 21858663. Epub 2011/08/23. Eng).

56. Whitson PA, Pietrzyk RA, Jones JA, Nelman-Gonzalez M, Hudson EK, Sams CF. Effect of potassium citrate therapy on the risk of renal stone formation during spaceflight. J Urol. 2009 Nov;182(5):2490–6. (PubMed PMID: 19765769. Epub 2009/09/22. Eng).

# Chapter 10
# Thiazides and Calcium Stones: Overrated or Underused?

John J. Knoedler and Amy E. Krambeck

## Introduction

The incidence of stone disease ranges from 10 to 15 % in a lifetime, with a higher predilection for adult men than women [1, 2]. Annual cost for stone disease in the USA is estimated to be greater than US$ 2 billion and rising, despite increasing outpatient management [2]. In the expanding era of health cost management, preventative measures for chronic diseases have appropriately come under increasing scrutiny. With the high recurrence rate among stone formers, the prevention of recurrent stone disease provides opportunity to improve not only patient care but also to contain cost by curbing the need for acute intervention for symptomatic stones.

Calcium-based stones represent the most common form, at over 60 % of all stones [1]. Thiazide-type diuretics have been in use for decades to not only treat hypertension, but as prevention for recurrent calcium stones. Well tolerated, relatively inexpensive, and with randomized, controlled trials to support their use [3–12], thiazides have been a workhorse of stone prevention. However, with further understanding of the complex nature of stone disease, and increasing evidence to support the effectiveness of dietary measures and alternative medical therapies, the value of thiazides for the prevention of recurrent calcium nephrolithiasis has recently come into question. Do thiazides remain the appropriate gold standard for stone prevention, and are thus underused, or are they in fact overrated? This chapter will explore the rational for thiazide usage in the prevention of recurrent calcium stone disease, evaluate the evidence in favor of and against thiazides as first-line therapy, and finally examine the cost-effective use of thiazides and their comparative effectiveness to alternative forms of treatment.

A. E. Krambeck (✉) · J. J. Knoedler
Department of Urology, Mayo Clinic, 200 1st St., SW, Rochester, MN 55905, USA
e-mail: krambeck.amy@mayo.edu

M. S. Pearle, S. Y. Nakada (eds.), *Practical Controversies in Medical Management of Stone Disease,* DOI 10.1007/978-1-4614-9575-8_10,

© Springer Science+Business Media New York 2014

"

**Table 10.1** Typical findings among varying types of hypercalciuria

|  | Serum calcium | Parathyroid | Urinary calcium (fasting) | Treatments |
|---|---|---|---|---|
| Absorptive | Normal | ↓ | Normal | Calcium binders (no longer used) Thiazides Potassium citrate |
| Renal leak | Normal | ↑ | ↑ | Thiazides Potassium citrate |
| Resorptive | ↑ | ↑ | ↑ | Treat underlying cause of elevate PTH |

# Pathophysiology of Calcium Stone Disease: A Brief Review

Calcium homeostasis in the body, as well as the urine, is a complex multifactorial system with many variables impacting normal function. Though a thorough discussion of the pathophysiology of calcium stone disease is beyond the scope of this chapter, a brief review is appropriate. The most common urinary finding in recurrent stone formers is hypercalciuria, and as such is often the target of therapy such as thiazide diuretics [1]. Additional major factors contributing to the formation of calcium stones include urinary oxalate, citrate, uric acid, and urine pH [1]. When an imbalance of the urinary milieu occurs, nucleation and subsequent stone formation is the result. The goal of medical therapy for recurrent stone formers is to bring the urinary profile into a more favorable alignment to prevent stone formation such as reducing urinary calcium, increasing urinary citrate, improving urinary pH, or reducing hyperuricosuria.

## *Types of Hypercalciuria*

Hypercalciuria is frequently implicated in calcium-stone formation, and indeed the treatment of hypercalciuria has been shown to reduce stone-formation rates regardless of the underlying cause. Hypercalciuria may be separated into three main types: absorptive hypercalciuria, renal leak hypercalciuria, and resorptive hypercalciuria [1, 13, 14]. Table 10.1 shows the various types of hypercalciuria, and their classic metabolic findings. Absorptive hypercalciuria represents the most common form, and results from increased intestinal absorption of calcium. By definition absorptive hypercalciuria is diagnosed by an increase in urinary calcium excretion >2.0 mg/ mg creatinine after an oral calcium load [1]. Due to the increased absorption, parathyroid function is often suppressed, though serum-calcium levels are typically normal. Absorptive hypercalciuria is further classified as type I, type II, and renal phosphate leak [1]. Type I absorptive is unresponsive to dietary changes, whereas in type II absorptive urinary calcium normalizes with a low calcium diet. Finally, in renal phosphate leak absorptive hypercalciuria, increased stimulation of vitamin D from low plasma phosphate leads to an increase in intestinal absorption. In contrast, renal leak hypercalciuria is defined by a persistent elevated urinary calcium level despite fasting [1]. Due to the persistent calcium drain, the parathyroid is stimulated, and secondary hyperparathyroidism results. As a result, significant bone reabsorption may occur leading to osteopenia. Historically, calcium binders such as sodium cellulose phosphate have been used for absorptive hypercalciuria, while thiazides have been used for renal leak hypercalciuria [1]. However, due to side effects, calcium binders are no longer used and thiazides are employed for absorptive hypercalciuria as well. Finally, resorptive hypercalciuria is a relatively rare cause of hypercalciuria and results from primary hyperparathyroidism. Bone loss can be significant with resorptive hypercalciuria, but the condition is corrected with removal of the offending parathyroid glands.

## Pro Arguments: The Use of Thiazides in Calcium Stone Prevention

### Thiazides: Pharmacologic Mechanism of Action and Rational for Use

As early as 1959, researchers noticed the impact of thiazide diuretics on decreasing calcium excretion in the urine [15]. Thiazide diuretics function in the proximal and distal convoluted tubule by inhibiting the Na-Cl cotransporter. Inhibition of the transporter results in loss of sodium in the urine and a volume-contracted state. To compensate for the volume contraction, the kidney will passively reabsorb sodium and calcium in the proximal convoluted tubules, thereby decreasing urinary concentrations of calcium. Thiazide diuretics also increase reabsorption of calcium in the distal tubule through activation of the sodium/calcium ATPase antiporter. Loss of urinary sodium activates the antiporter, which leads to more calcium in the interstitium and a lower intracellular calcium concentration. The low intracellular concentration of calcium results in greater diffusion of calcium from the urine into the cells by passive transport. Although both mechanisms are highly effective at lowering urinary calcium, the effect of the thiazide diuretic can be completely negated by large amounts of sodium in the urine. Thus, to achieve the maximal hypocalciuric effect of thiazide diuretics the patient must be kept on a low sodium diet, generally around 2–2.5 g per day.

While decreasing urinary calcium levels, thiazides are known to cause hypokalemia leading to the absorption of citrate; a potent inhibitor of stone formation [14]. The hypocitraturic effect is primarily mediated by an intracellular acidosis induced by hypokalemia, with resultant inhibition of citrate excretion. Thus, when thiazides are prescribed, they are often given in conjunction with a potassium chloride or potassium citrate supplementation to negate the hypokalemic effects [13, 14]. Another strategy, which avoids potassium supplementation, is to prescribe thiazides with ACE inhibitors to limit the thiazide hypokalemic effect. In addition to alterations

**Table 10.2** Randomized, controlled trials for thiazide-type diuretics in stone prevention [3–12]

| Year | Author | Treatment/dose | Outcome (RR) |
|---|---|---|---|
| 1981 | Brocks et al. | Bendroflumethiazide 2.5 mg TID | None |
| 1982 | Schloz et al. | HCTZ 25 mg BID | None |
| 1984 | Laerum et al. | HCTZ 25 mg BID | 0.39 |
| 1984 | Wilson et al. | HCTZ 100 mg QD | 0.48 |
| 1985 | Robertson et al. | Bendroflumethiazide 2.5 mg TID | 0.38 |
| 1986 | Mortenson et al. | Bendroflumethiazide 2.5 mg TID | None |
| 1988 | Ettinger et al. | Chlorthalidone | 0.23 |
| 1992 | Ohkawa et al. | Trichlormethiazide 4 mg | 0.42 |
| 1993 | Borghi et al. | Indapamide 2.5 mg daily | 0.21 |
| 2006 | Fernandez-Rodrigue et al. | HCTZ 50 mg QD | 0.56 |

in potassium metabolism, thiazides have a hyperuricemic effect, attributed to increased, proximal tubule sodium reabsorption and subsequent urate reabsorption. The increase in serum urate is typically clinically insignificant and does not require treatment [16].

As an alternative to hydrochlorothiazide, thiazide-like diuretics (indapamide and chlorthalidone) induce a similar hypocalciuric effect and have been shown effective in treating calcium stones [9, 11]. While similarly effective to traditional thiazides, these thiazide-like diuretics have the advantage of once daily dosing as opposed to multiple times per day for thiazides. Whether utilizing thiazides or thiazide-type diuretics, clinicians historically have found that the diuretics lose efficacy over time, and a thiazide "holiday" is needed periodically. However, in the 2009 Cochrane review of pharmacologic interventions for hypercalciuria, thiazides were shown to maintain efficacy for a period of at least 36 months, and no time frame for decreased efficacy was identified [17]. Therefore, the use of thiazide "holidays" remains controversial and is at the clinician's discretion.

## *Efficacy of Thiazides for Prevention of Calcium Urolithiasis*

A recent 2009 Cochrane review entitled, "Pharmacologic interventions for preventing complications in idiopathic hypercalciuria," examined the evidence-based role of various interventions on calcium stone formation and complications [17]. Reviewing four randomized, controlled trials including a total of 285 patients, thiazide diuretics were found, along with dietary control, to result in an approximately 60% decrease in patients with a recurrence of urolithiasis (RR 1.61, 95% CI 1.33–1.96), as well as a decrease in the number of stones per patient per year (mean difference −0.18, 95% CI −0.30 to −0.06) [17]. Furthermore, the review found that the hypocalciuric effect of thiazides is maintained for at least 3 years [17].

To date, at least ten randomized, controlled trials have evaluated the use of thiazide-type diuretics for the prevention of recurrent calcium urolithiasis (Table 10.2). The clinical trials on thiazide-type diuretics have a large degree of heterogeneity between them, but nonetheless they appear to be effective. It is interesting to note that the beneficial impact of thiazides was found even in studies where hypercalciuria was not among the inclusion criteria, indicating the protective effect of thiazides may in fact be maintained regardless of urinary calcium levels [18]. Pearle et al., in 1999, performed a meta-analysis of medical prevention for calcium oxalate nephrolithiasis [19]. In the meta-analysis the authors analyzed all available data for treatments, evaluated as an aggregate, to assess whether treatment as a whole with any form of medication significantly impacted stone recurrence. The impact of each individual treatment (including thiazides type diuretics, allopurinol, phosphate, magnesium and alkali citrates) was then evaluated to determine the impact on symptomatic stone recurrence. A statistically significant ($p=0.04$) benefit for intervention, driven largely by the benefit derived from thiazide diuretics ($p=0.02$), was noted [19]. While other therapies (including citrate therapy) may in fact be beneficial, conclusive data is currently lacking based on the current study.

Due to the hypokalemic effect of thiazides and the subsequent acidosis with decrease in urinary citrate, many clinicians routinely employ citrate therapy concurrently with thiazides. Of the randomized, controlled trials to date included in the 2009 Cochrane Review, one compared thiazide usage alone and in combination with potassium citrate [17]. Though not statistically significant, the combination therapy appeared to decrease the recurrence. However, the value of citrate therapy in combination with thiazides has yet to be studied in a large, randomized, controlled trial.

## *Evidenced-Based Use of Thiazides*

To date, ten randomized, controlled trials have looked at the impact of thiazide diuretics on preventing urolithiasis [3–6]. While high-level evidence exists for the use of thiazides in the prevention of urolithiasis, clinicians often employ dosages not studied in randomized, controlled trials. Over the past decades, the typical dosage of HCTZ used for hypertension is 12.5 –25 mg daily. Such dosages, however, have yet to be studied with high-level evidence. In the randomized, controlled trials to date, the doses of thiazide-type medications used were indapamide 2.5 mg/day, chlorthalidone 25–50 mg/day, HCTZ 50–100 mg/daily [17, 18]. Vigen et al., in a multi-center review of 107 patients treated with thiazide-type diuretics for calcium-containing stones, found that among those being prescribed HCTZ ($n=102$) only 35 % were prescribed dosages of $\geq 50$ mg/day, with 52 % receiving 25 mg/day and 13 % receiving 12.5 mg/day [20]. Furthermore, in an analyzed subset of six patients, increasing the dosage from 25 to 50 mg/day decreased 24 h urinary calcium ($p=0.051$) [20]. Though common to use low-dose thiazides for the treatment of hypertension, such dosages lack clinical evidence for the prevention of hypercalciuria. In fact, modest evidence suggests that hypocalciuric benefits may occur in a dose-dependent relationship.

Another potential benefit of thiazide and thiazide-like diuretics is their effects on bone density. Hypercalciuria, regardless of the presence of stone disease, is associated with bone loss, and this difference may be more pronounced among stone formers [21, 22]. A recent Cochrane review found evidence that thiazides may prevent osteoporosis based on limited series, but to date no randomized, controlled trials have evaluated this endpoint.

## Con Arguments Against Thiazides for Calcium Stone Disease: Alternative Cause Theory and the Side Effects of Thiazides

### *Hypocitraturia*

The rationale for thiazides as prevention for recurrent calcium stone disease is based largely upon the belief that hypercalciuria is the driving factor in recurrent stone disease. Alternatively, citrate therapy is often touted as a catchall first-line therapy for recurrent nephrolithiasis. Urinary citrate prevents stone formation by a number of mechanisms, including forming a complex with calcium in the renal tubule, thus limiting the available calcium for nucleation [23]. Additionally, citrate prevents the agglomeration of calcium to existing crystals, further inhibiting stone formation [23]. While citrate therapy shows benefit for the prevention of calcium stones in the presence of hypercalciuria as well as hypocitraturia, citrate further improves outcomes in patients who have hyperuricosuria in the presence of calcium nephrolithiasis, and may thus alleviate the need to add allopurinol to a thiazide regimen in these patients [24]. For these reasons, advocates of citrate therapy frequently point to it as a "one-stop-shop" for stone prevention; citrate therapy may be adequate first-line therapy for most calcium-based stone formers.

### *Adverse Effects of Thiazides*

Though thiazide-type diuretics are generally well tolerated, and frequently employed for both stone disease and hypertension, metabolic side effects may occur, possibly limiting their efficacy (Table 10.3 lists side effects and contraindications to thiazides). Huen and Goldfarb performed a review of the literature including nine randomized, controlled trials to assess the metabolic effect of thiazides and their potential impact among patients with stones [16]. Among the nine randomized, controlled trials included, the authors found a paucity of data regarding the metabolic impact of thiazides. Two studies included lipid and glucose levels (without significant changes), and three measured potassium with two of those identifying significant changes in serum potassium levels, while the third did not [16]. The

**Table 10.3** Side effects and contraindications of thiazides

| | |
|---|---|
| Relative contraindications | Pregnancy |
| | Hypersensitivity reaction to thiazides |
| | Sulfa allergy (risk of cross-reactivity) |
| Side effects | Orthostasis and hypotension |
| | Glucose intolerance |
| | Hyperlipidemia |
| | Hyperkalemia |
| | Hypercalcemia |
| | Gout precipitated by hyperuricemia |

authors concluded that the lack of robust data regarding the adverse metabolic impact of thiazides among recurrent stone formers leaves this question largely unanswered.

Interestingly, Huen and Goldfarb note the findings of the Antihypertensive and Lipid-Lowering Treatment to Prevent Heart Attack Trial (ALLHAT), notably their impact on potassium via thiazide-induced hypokalemia, impacts on glucose tolerance, and altered lipid profiles [16, 25]. ALLHAT followed over 30,000 patients age 55 or older who had hypertension and at least one other coronary heart disease risk factor, and randomized them to angiotensin-converting enzyme inhibitor, calcium channel blocker, or diuretic therapy, with primary outcome of myocardial infarction [25]. On subset analysis, the authors analyzed the metabolic impact of thiazides among this specific population. Thiazides increased the risk of hypokalemia, elevated LDL and triglycerides, and glucose intolerance. In fact, patients treated with chlorthalidone had an increased rate of new-onset diabetes at 4 years of follow-up compared to patients treated with amlodipine or lisinopril [16, 25]. These findings were confirmed by the Nurses Health Study and Health Professional Studies, where thiazides for treatment of hypertension increased the risk of new-onset diabetes on multivariate analysis [16]. Though the population of patients treated for hypertension with thiazides represents a distinct population from those treated for nephrolithiasis, nonetheless the data provide insight into the potential long-term effect of thiazide usage. Given the significant lack of data on adverse effects of thiazide-type diuretics used for the prevention of recurrent stones, further research is needed to define outcomes and risk.

Among patients with hyperuricemia and a gouty diathesis in the presence of calcium stones, treatment of uricemia with allopurinol has the potential to be beneficial in preventing calcium stones since uric acid reduces the solubility of calcium in the urine [17, 26]. Thiazides may also induce uric acid reabsorption and hyperuricemia, which has been thought to be of limited clinical significance [16, 27]. However, in a prospective analysis of over 45,000 patients without prior history of gout, the usage of diuretics (including thiazides) resulted in a 77 % increased risk of new incidence of gout [27]. Therefore, patients initiating treatment with thiazide-type diuretics should undergo periodic evaluation of serum uric acid levels, and monitoring for the development of gout.

## Economics of Thiazides: Cost-Effectiveness in the Treatment of Calcium Stones

While the value to the individual patient of remaining stone free cannot truly be quantified, the economics of medical management of stone disease play an important role in the decision to evaluate and treat urolithiasis patients. Particularly in this changing era of medical cost and payment restructuring, such assessments will undoubtedly become increasingly important. Which patients benefit from metabolic evaluation and prophylaxis? Is an abbreviated metabolic analysis sufficient, and to what degree does the subsequent treatment prevent stones and thus contain cost? Furthermore, as treatment for stone events becomes increasingly efficient, how does the long-term cost of prophylaxis compare to treatment for acute episodes? These questions will continue to shape the debate on the treatment of recurrent stone disease. While an in-depth discussion of the economics of stones disease is beyond the scope of this chapter, we will review the pertinent points with regards to prophylaxis with thiazides.

Lotan and Pearle, in their review entitled, "Economics of Stone Management," examine the salient points of medical management for urolithiasis [28]. As the authors point out, defining the economic burden of stone disease is difficult, particularly in the more abstract US payer system. Indeed, while the term "cost" is often used interchangeably with "charge," the true cost to the system often (or usually) is not reflected in the charge applied for services. Though the authors identified a great deal of heterogeneity in study design, from a purely cost-based perspective, conservative management represents the most cost-effective treatment for not only first-time stone formers, but for recurrent stone formers as well. However, with minimal evaluation and either directed or empiric drug therapy a somewhat modest rise in cost may result in a clinically significant decrease in stone recurrence [28, 29].

While Lotan and Pearle found that conservative therapy was most cost-effective across the board, they also note that among patients being worked up with metabolic evaluation and treatment, a simple metabolic evaluation was more cost effective than a complete metabolic evaluation with rather comparable efficacy at stone prevention [28, 29]. However, among recurrent stone formers, empiric therapy with potassium citrate was nearly as effective, and less costly than even a simple metabolic evaluation and treatment. These findings highlight the fact that, even among recurrent stone formers, a minimalist approach to evaluation and treatment may represent the most prudent approach from both a cost-effective and stone-free point of view. A more in-depth analysis might then be reserved for the complex patients who are refractory to initial evaluation and treatment. Among first-time stone formers, a conservative approach perhaps with lifestyle and dietary changes (i.e., increasing fluid intake) may suffice.

## *Comparative Effectiveness of Thiazides, Diet/Lifestyle Modifications, and Alternative Pharmacotherapy*

While thiazide-based therapy is effective for the prevention of stones, less defined is the comparative effectiveness of thiazides with both conservative lifestyle interventions, as well alternative medical therapies. However, recent studies have sought to clarify this difference. In 2009, a consortium of authors performed a review of dietary, fluid intake, and supplements for the prevention of urolithiasis [30]. A significant benefit was noted with fluid intake of 2 L/day or of a volume to maintain >2.5 L of urine output per day. Additionally, the evidence supported the decreased intake of soft drinks, as well as promoting regular calcium intake [30]. The regular intake of dietary calcium is felt to bind to oxalate in the GI tract, and prevent hyperoxaluria.

In a 2013 review of 28 randomized, controlled trials, Fink et al. reviewed the available evidence for treatment of nephrolithiasis [31]. They found that simply increasing fluid intake will halve the risk for subsequent stone formation, and may be appropriate as the only intervention for first-time stone formers. Furthermore, the reduction of intake of soft drinks with phosphoric acid among those who had a high baseline intake further reduced risk of stone formation. Interestingly, there was inconclusive evidence to support other dietary interventions. With regard to medical interventions, thiazides, citrate therapy, and allopurinol all decreased the risk of recurrent stone formation. Among the studies reviewed, a significant benefit of combination therapy (i.e., thiazide plus citrate therapy as opposed to thiazides alone) was not identified, with one notable exception; among patients with calcium stones and hyperuricosuria or hyperuricemia, the addition of allopurinol to thiazides significantly reduced the risk of subsequent stone formation [31]. The authors conclude that increased fluid intake alone or in combination with a decrease in soft drink consumption may be adequate in first-time stone formers. However, for recurrent formers who have increased fluid intake, thiazides, citrate therapy, and allopurinol all show benefit for prevention of recurrent stones [31].

## Summary of Evidence and Conclusion

Thiazide diuretics represent perhaps the most robustly studied intervention for recurrent calcium-based stones, with significant clinical evidence to support their use. Thiazides and thiazide-like diuretics are typically well tolerated, with minimal adverse effects. For recurrent calcium-based stone formers with hypercalciuria, thiazides represent an appropriate first-line choice after a limited metabolic evaluation. Though ultimately not as cost-effective as conservative therapy or empiric therapy for even recurrent stone formers, thiazide diuretics represent a reasonable middle ground where the small increase in cost may justify the added improvement in stone-free rates. However, the evidence indicates that clinicians routinely fail to use thiazides in an evidenced-based fashion, often employing lower doses than have been included prospective studies. While lower doses are routinely used for hypertensive patients and may in fact be appropriate for the prevention of stones in order to decrease side effects and increase compliance, data on their use for the prevention of recurrent calcium stones are lacking. Furthermore, implementation of a low-sodium diet is paramount in producing the hypocalciuric effects of thiazide diuretics

Among first-time stone formers, conservative therapy with minimal lifestyle interventions, such as increased fluid intake, are likely sufficient. Among recurrent stone formers, a limited metabolic evaluation with treatment is warranted. In such a role, thiazide-type diuretics are effective and likely underused. With hypercalciuria representing the most common urinary risk factor among stone formers, thiazide usage as first-line therapy to correct the imbalance is appropriate. Though studies suggest that the addition of citrate therapy to thiazides does not improve stone-free rates, the level of evidence is low and the use of potassium citrate to offset the secondary hypokalemia and resultant acidosis that can occur with thiazide usage may be appropriate. Additionally, among patients with hyperuricemia and/or hyperuricosuria in the setting of recurrent calcium stones, the addition of allopurinol to a first-line thiazide regimen may be beneficial. Nonetheless, thiazide diuretics with or without a secondary medication are effective prophylaxis against recurrent calcium nephrolithiasis with high-level evidence to support their use. As such, thiazide diuretics should remain the gold standard for treatment.

# References


1. Wein AJ, Kavoussi LR, Novick AC, Partin AW, Peters CA, editors. Campbell-walsh urology. 10th ed. Philadelphia: Saunders Elsevier; 2012.
2. Pearle MS, Calhoun EA, Curhan GC. Urologic diseases in America project: urolithiasis. J Urol. 2005;173(3):848–57.
3. Brocks P, Dahl C, Wolf H, Transbøl I. Do thiazides prevent recurrent idiopathic renal calcium stones? Lancet. 1981;2(8238):124–5.
4. Scholz D, Schwille PO, Sigel A. Double-blind study with thiazide in recurrent calcium lithiasis. J Urol. 1982;128(5):903–7.
5. Laerum E, Larsen S. Thiazide prophylaxis of urolithiasis. A double-blind study in general practice. Acta Med Scand. 1984;215(4):383–9.
6. Wilson D, Strauss A, Manuel M. Comparison of medical treatments for the prevention of recurrent calcium nephrolithiasis. Urol Res. 1984;12:39–40.
7. Robertson WG, Peacock M, Selby PL, Williams RE, Clark P, Chisholm GD, et al. A multicentre trial to evaluate three treatments for recurrent idiopathic calcium stone disease—a preliminary report. In: Schwille PO, Smith LH, Robertson WG, Vahlensieck W, editors. Urolithiasis and related clinical research. New York: Plenum Press; 1985.p. 545–8.
8. Mortensen JT, Schultz A, Ostergaard AH. Thiazides in the prophylactic treatment of recurrent idiopathic kidney stones. Int Urol Nephrol. 1986;18(3):265–9.
9. Ettinger B, Citron JT, Livermore B, Dolman LI. Chlorthalidone reduces calcium oxalate calculous recurrence but magnesium hydroxide does not. J Urol. 1988;139(4):679–84.
10. Ohkawa M, Tokunaga S, Nakashima T, Orito M, Hisazumi H. Thiazide treatment for calcium urolithiasis in patients with idiopathic hypercalciuria. Br J Urol. 1992;69(6):571–6.

11. Borghi L, Meschi T, Guerra A, Novarini A. Randomized prospective study of a nonthiazide diuretic, indapamide, in preventing calcium stone recurrences. J Cardiovasc Pharmacol. 1993;22(6):78–86.
12. Fernández-Rodríguez A, Arrabal-Martín M, García-Ruiz MJ, Arrabal-Polo MA, Pichardo-Pichardo S, Zuluaga-Gómez A. Papel de las tiazidas en la profilaxis de la litiasis cálcica recidivante. Actas Urológicas Españolas. 2006;30:305–9.
13. Park S, Pearle MS. Pathophysiology and management of calcium stones. Urol Clin North Am. 2007;34(3):323–34.
14. Pak CY. Pharmacotherapy of kidney stones. Expert Opin Pharmacother. 2008;9(9):1509–18.
15. Lamberg BA, Kuhlback B. Effect of chlorothiazide and hydrochlorothiazide on the excretion of calcium in urine. Scand J Clin Lab Invest. 1959;11:351–7.
16. Huen SC, Goldfarb DS. Adverse metabolic side effects of thiazides: implications for patients with calcium nephrolithiasis. J Urol. 2007;177(4):1238–43.
17. Escribano J, Balaguer A, Pagone F, Feliu A, Roqué I, Figuls M. Pharmacological interventions for preventing complications in idiopathic hypercalciuria. Cochrane Database Syst Rev. 2009 Jan 21;(1):CD004754.
18. Reilly RF, Peixoto AJ, Desir GV. The evidence-based use of thiazide diuretics in hypertension and nephrolithiasis. Clin J Am Soc Nephrol. 2010;5(10):1893–1903.
19. Pearle MS, Roehrborn CG, Pak CY. Meta-analysis of randomized trials for medical prevention of calcium oxalate nephrolithiasis. J Endourol. 1999;13(9):679–85.
20. Vigen R, Weideman R, Reilly R. Thiazides diuretics in the treatment of nephrolithiasis: are we using them in an evidence-based fashion? Int Urol Nephrol. 2011;43(3):813–9.
21. Asplin JR, Bauer KA, Kinder J, Müller G, Coe BJ, Parks JH, et al. Bone mineral density and urine calcium excretion among subjects with and without nephrolithiasis. Kidney Int. 2003;63(2):662–9.
22. Asplin JR, Donahue S, Kinder J, Coe FL. Urine calcium excretion predicts bone loss in idiopathic hypercalciuria. Kidney Int. 2006;70(8):1463–7.
23. de Cogain M, Krambeck A. Pathogenesis of stone disease. AUA Update Series. 2011;30(Lesson 3):25–31.
24. Pak CY, Peterson R. Successful treatment of hyperuricosuric calcium oxalate nephrolithiasis with potassium citrate. Arch Intern Med. 1986;146(5):863–7.
25. ALLHAT Officers and Coordinators for the ALLHAT Collaborative Research Group. The Antihypertensive and lipid-lowering treatment to prevent heart attack trial. Major outcomes in high-risk hypertensive patients randomized to angiotensin-converting enzyme inhibitor or calcium channel blocker vs diuretic: the antihypertensive and lipid-lowering treatment to prevent heart attack trial (ALLHAT). JAMA. 2002;288(23):2981–97.
26. Eisner BH, Goldfarb DS, Pareek G. Pharmacologic treatment of kidney stone disease. Urol Clin North Am. 2013;40(1):21–30.
27. Choi HK, Atkinson K, Karlson EW, Curhan G. Obesity, weight change, hypertension, diuretic use, and risk of gout in men: the health professionals follow-up study. Arch Intern Med. 2005;165(7):742–8.
28. Lotan Y, Pearle MS. Economics of stone management. Urol Clin North Am. 2007;34(3):443–53.
29. Lotan Y, Cadeddu JA, Roerhborn CG, Pak CY, Pearle MS. Cost-effectiveness of medical management strategies for nephrolithiasis. J Urol. 2004;172(6 Pt 1):2275–81.
30. Fink HA, Akornor JW, Garimella PS, MacDonald R, Cutting A, Rutks IR, et al. Diet, fluid, or supplements for secondary prevention of nephrolithiasis: a systematic review and meta-analysis of randomized trials. European Urology. 2009;56(1):72–80.
31. Fink HA, Wilt TJ, Eidman KE, Garimella PS, MacDonald R, Rutks IR, et al. Medical management to prevent recurrent nephrolithiasis in adults: a systematic review for an American College of Physicians Clinical Guideline. Ann Inter Med. 2013;158(7):535–43.

# Index



M. S. Pearle, S. Y. Nakada (eds.), *Practical Controversies in Medical Management
of Stone Disease,* DOI 10.1007/978-1-4614-9575-8,
© Springer Science+Business Media New York 2014